V VETERINARY
M MEDICAL
S SCHOOL
A ADMISSION
R REQUIREMENTS

VETERINARY MEDICAL SCHOOL ADMISSION REQUIREMENTS

2006 Edition for 2007 Matriculation

Association of American
Veterinary Medical Colleges

PURDUE UNIVERSITY PRESS   WEST LAFAYETTE, INDIANA

Compiled by the Association of American Veterinary Medical Colleges;
Michael Peart and Shaba Lightfoot, editors

Printed in the United States of America

ISBN 1-55753-423-3
        978-1-55753-423-1

ISSN 1089-6465

CONTENTS

ABBREVIATIONS

AAVMC	Association of American Veterinary Medical Colleges
AVMA	American Veterinary Medical Association
BA/BS	Bachelor of Arts or Bachelor of Science degrees
CLEP	College Level Examination Program
CVMA	Canadian Veterinary Medical Association
DVM/VMD	Doctor of Veterinary Medicine degree
GRE®	Graduate Record Examination
MCAT	Medical College Admission Test
MS	Master of Science degree
PhD	Doctor of Philosophy degree
SREB	Southern Regional Education Board
TOEFL	Test of English as a Foreign Language
VMCAS	Veterinary Medical College Application Service
VMD/DVM	Veterinary Medical Doctor degree
VMSAR	Veterinary Medical School Admission Requirements
WICHE	Western Interstate Commission for Higher Education

Veterinary Medicine: Choices and Challenges

Considered from the perspective of comparative medicine, veterinarians help animals and people live longer, healthier lives. They serve society by preventing and treating animal disease, improving the quality of the environment, ensuring the safety of food, controlling diseases transmitted from animals, and advancing medical knowledge. The Doctor of Veterinary Medicine degree can lead to diverse career opportunities and different lifestyles from a solo mixed-animal practice in a rural area to a teaching or research position at an urban university, medical center, or industrial laboratory. The majority of veterinarians in the United States are in private practice, although significant numbers are involved in preventive medicine, regulatory veterinary medicine, military veterinary medicine, laboratory animal medicine, research and development in industry, and teaching and research in a variety of basic science and clinical disciplines.

License to Practice

The DVM (or VMD) degree is awarded after 4 years of successful study at an accredited college of veterinary medicine. Graduate veterinarians are eligible to apply for a license to practice. Licensing is controlled by states and provinces, each of which has rules and procedures for legal practice within its own jurisdiction. All require satisfactory completion of the national board examination, and most have other requirements, including additional tests and interviews.

Specialization

Veterinarians may choose to become specialists in a clinical area or to work with particular species. The first step on the path toward specialization is usually an internship.

Internship

Internships are 1-year programs in either small- or large-animal medicine and surgery. The most prestigious internship programs are at veterinary medical colleges or at very large private veterinary hospitals with board-certified veterinarians on staff. Since internships are usually at large referral centers, interns are exposed to a larger number of challenging cases than they would be likely to see in a smaller private practice.

Veterinary students in their senior year and veterinary graduates apply for

1

internships through a matching program. Internship applicants and training hospitals rank each other in order of preference, and a computerized system matches each applicant with the highest-ranking teaching hospital that ranked the applicant. Academic performance in the veterinary professional curriculum, as well as recommendations from veterinary school faculty, is considered in the ranking of internship applicants.

Most veterinary interns in the United States receive a nominal salary, and their educational debts, if any, may be postponed in some governmentally subsidized loan programs. Veterinarians can often command a higher starting salary in private practice after completion of an internship. Also, an internship is the next step, after receiving the DVM degree, toward residency and board certification.

Residency Training

Veterinarians who complete internships or who have 2 years of private-practice experience are eligible to apply for residency programs. Residency training is more specialized than an internship. Currently, residency training is available in internal medicine, surgery, cardiology, dermatology, ophthalmology, exotic small animal medicine, pathology, neurology, radiology, anesthesiology, and oncology. The programs take 2 to 3 years to complete, depending on the nature of the specialty. Successful completion of a residency is required for certification by any of the veterinary medical specialty boards. Some residencies combine research and graduate study to lead to a master's degree.

Board Certification

Veterinary board certification and diplomate status are available for 20 specialties: anesthesiology, animal behavior, clinical pharmacology, dentistry, dermatology, emergency and critical care, internal medicine, laboratory animal medicine, microbiology, nutrition, ophthalmology, pathology, poultry medicine, private practice, preventive medicine, radiology, surgery, theriogenology (reproduction), toxicology, and zoological medicine.

Private and Public Practice

A significant percentage of veterinary graduates are engaged in private practice, either as an owner of a solo practice or, more likely, as a partner or associate in a group practice. Increasingly, veterinarians work together as a team, which allows a wider range of services to be provided.

Small-animal veterinarians focus their efforts primarily on dogs and cats but are seeing a growing number of pet birds and exotic animals such as reptiles.

Veterinarians specializing in large animals often place their emphasis on horses, cattle, or pigs, and work both on a farm-call and an in-clinic basis. A mixed-animal veterinarian works with all types of animals.

Some veterinarians obtain further specialization in such areas as diseases or disorders of the eyes of cats or reproduction difficulties in cattle.

Public practice provides a variety of opportunities at the national, state, county, or city levels. Opportunities in food safety, public health, the military, animal disease control, research, and the care and maintenance of wildlife abound.

Industry

Veterinarians have many opportunities available to them in private industry, particularly in the fields of nutrition and pharmaceuticals. Assisting in the development of new products in the animal industry, conducting research for pharmaceutical companies, diagnosing disease and drug effects as pathologists, or safeguarding the health of laboratory animal colonies are all interesting career possibilities. Some veterinarians may be employed by zoos and aquariums and may act as consultants to wildlife preservation groups, game farms, or fisheries.

New or Unusual Career Opportunities

By the very nature of the many species of animals involved and the wide variety of clientele served, the opportunities available to today's veterinarian are abun-

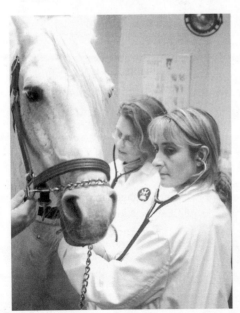

dant. The role of the veterinarian in society has changed and evolved over time, so that they are now specially qualified to take part in many problems related to the environment, local community health, food resource management, zoo animal care, space and marine biology, and wildlife preservation.

A Tufts University Cummings School of Veterinary Medicine student checks out a horse with advice from her professor. Photo courtesy of Andy Cunningham of the Tufts University Cummings School of Veterinary Medicine.

ALPHABETICAL LISTING OF VETERINARY SCHOOLS

United States

Auburn University	Auburn University, Alabama
California, University of	Davis, California
Colorado State University	Fort Collins, Colorado
Cornell University	Ithaca, New York
Florida, University of	Gainesville, Florida
Georgia, University of	Athens, Georgia
Illinois, University of	Urbana, Illinois
Iowa State University	Ames, Iowa
Kansas State University	Manhattan, Kansas
Louisiana State University	Baton Rouge, Louisiana
Michigan State University	East Lansing, Michigan
Minnesota, University of	St. Paul, Minnesota
Mississippi State University	Mississippi State, Mississippi
Missouri, University of	Columbia, Missouri
North Carolina State University	Raleigh, North Carolina
Ohio State University	Columbus, Ohio
Oklahoma State University	Stillwater, Oklahoma
Oregon State University	Corvallis, Oregon
Pennsylvania, University of	Philadelphia, Pennsylvania
Purdue University	West Lafayette, Indiana
Tennessee, University of	Knoxville, Tennessee
Texas A & M University	College Station, Texas
Tufts University	North Grafton, Massachusetts
Tuskegee University	Tuskegee, Alabama
Virginia-Maryland Regional College of Veterinary Medicine	Blacksburg, Virginia
Washington State University	Pullman, Washington
Wisconsin, University of	Madison, Wisconsin
Western University of Health Sciences	Pomona, California

International

Edinburgh, University of	Edinburgh, Scotland
Glasgow, University of	Glasgow, Scotland
Guelph, University of	Guelph, Ontario, Canada
Massey University	Palmerston North, New Zealand
Montréal, Université de	Montréal, Québec, Canada
Prince Edward Island, University of	Charlottetown, Prince Edward Island, Canada
Saskatchewan, University of	Saskatoon, Saskatchewan, Canada

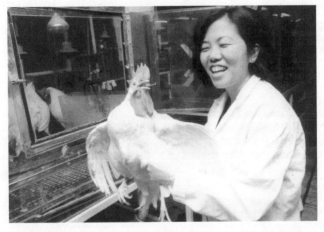

A student specializing in avian medicine examines a chicken as part of her study. Photo by Joey Rodgers, courtesy of University of Georgia College of Veterinary Medicine.

GEOGRAPHICAL LISTING OF VETERINARY SCHOOLS AND DIRECTORY OF ADMISSIONS OFFICES

United States

Alabama

Office for Academic Affairs
College of Veterinary Medicine
217 Goodwin Student Center
Auburn University
Auburn University AL 36849-5536

Office of Veterinary Admissions
College of Veterinary Medicine,
    Nursing, and Allied Health
Tuskegee University
Tuskegee AL 36088

California

School of Veterinary Medicine
Office of the Dean-Student Programs
University of California
One Shields Avenue
Davis CA 95616

Western University of
    Health Sciences
Office of Admissions
College of Veterinary Medicine
309 East 2nd Street
Pomona CA 91766-1854

Colorado

Office of the Dean
College of Veterinary Medicine and
    Biomedical Sciences
1601 Campus Delivery
Colorado State University
Fort Collins CO 80523-1601

Florida

Admissions Office
College of Veterinary Medicine
P.O. Box 100125
University of Florida
Gainesville FL 32610-0125

Georgia

Office for Academic Affairs
College of Veterinary Medicine
The University of Georgia
Athens GA 30602-7372

Illinois

Office of Academic and Student Affairs
College of Veterinary Medicine
University of Illinois at Urbana-
    Champaign
2271G Veterinary Medicine Basic
    Sciences Building
2001 South Lincoln Avenue
Urbana IL 61802

Indiana

Student Services Office
School of Veterinary Medicine
625 Harrison Street
Purdue University
West Lafayette IN 47907-2026

Iowa

Office of Admissions
College of Veterinary Medicine
2270 Veterniary Medicince
Iowa State University
P.O. Box 3020
Ames IA 50010-3020

Kansas
Office of Admissions
College of Veterinary Medicine
101 Trotter Hall
Kansas State University
Manhattan KS 66506-5601

Louisiana
Office of Veterinary Student and
Academic Affairs
School of Veterinary Medicine
Louisiana State University
Baton Rouge LA 70803

Massachusetts
Office of Admissions
Cummings School of Veterinary
   Medicine
Tufts University
200 Westboro Road
North Grafton MA 01536

Michigan
Office of Admissions
College of Veterinary Medicine
F-104 Veterinary Medical Center
Michigan State University
East Lansing MI 48824-1316

Minnesota
Office of Student Affairs and
   Admissions
College of Veterinary Medicine
460 Veterinary Medical Center
1365 Gortner Avenue
University of Minnesota
St. Paul MN 55108

Mississippi
Office of Student Affairs
College of Veterinary Medicine
P.O. Box 6100
Mississippi State University
Mississippi State MS 39762

Missouri
Office of Academic Affairs
College of Veterinary Medicine
W203 Veterinary Medicine Building
University of Missouri-Columbia
Columbia MO 65211

New York
Office of DVM Admissions
College of Veterinary Medicine
S2-009 Schurman Hall
Cornell University
Ithaca NY 14853-6401

North Carolina
Student Services Office
College of Veterinary Medicine
4700 Hillsborough Street, Box 8401
North Carolina State University
Raleigh NC 27606

Ohio
Chairperson, Admissions Committee
College of Veterinary Medicine
Suite 127 Veterinary Medicine
   Academic Building
1900 Coffey Road
The Ohio State University
Columbus OH 43210-1089

Oklahoma
Office of Admissions
110 McElory Hall
Center for Veterinary Health Sciences
College of Veterinary Medicine
Oklahoma State University
Stillwater OK 74078-2003

Oregon
Office of the Dean
College of Veterinary Medicine
Oregon State University
200 Magruder Hall
Corvallis OR 97331-4801

Pennsylvania
Admissions Office
School of Veterinary Medicine
3800 Spruce Street
University of Pennsylvania
Philadelphia PA 19104-6044

Tennessee
Admissions Office
College of Veterinary Medicine
2407 River Drive
Room A-104-C
The University of Tennessee
Knoxville TN 37996-4550

Texas
Office of the Dean
College of Veterinary Medicine
and Biomedical Sciences
Texas A & M University
College Station TX 77843-4461

Virginia
Admissions Coordinator
Virginia-Maryland Regional College
of Veterinary Medicine
Blacksburg VA 24061

Washington
Office of Student Services
College of Veterinary Medicine
Washington State University
P.O. Box 647012
Pullman WA 99164-7012

Wisconsin
Office of Academic Affairs
School of Veterinary Medicine
2015 Linden Drive
University of Wisconsin-Madison
Madison WI 53706-1102

International

Canada
Montréal
Service des Admissions
Université de Montréal
C.P. 6205
Succursale Centre-Ville
Montréal Québec H3C 3T5
Canada

Ontario
Admissions Services
University Centre, Level 3
University of Guelph
Guelph Ontario N1G 2W1
Canada

Prince Edward Island
Registrar's Office
Atlantic Veterinary College
University of Prince Edward Island
550 University Avenue
Charlottetown PEI C1A 4P3
Canada

Saskatchewan
Admissions Office
Western College of Veterinary
Medicine
University of Saskatchewan
52 Campus Drive
Saskatoon Saskatchewan S7N 5B4
Canada

New Zealand
International Student Affairs
Massey University Veterinary School
Institute of Veterinary Animal and
  Bio-Medical Sciences
College of Sciences
Massey University
Private Bag 11-222
Palmerston North
New Zealand

Scotland
Admissions Officer
School Office
Royal (Dick) School of
  Veterinary Studies
The University of Edinburgh
Summerhall
Edinburgh EH9 1QH
Scotland

Admissions Officer and Student
Affairs Coordinator
University of Glasgow Veterinary
  School
Bearsden Road
Bearsden
Glasgow G61 1QH
Scotland

LISTING OF SCHOOLS ACCEPTING NONRESIDENT/NONCONTRACT APPLICATIONS

United States	Number of Positions Available
Auburn University	10 positions; U.S. citizens only.
University of California	Limited number of positions.
Colorado State University	Up to 32 positions; international applicants considered.
Cornell University	Up to 35 positions; international applicants considered.
University of Florida	Not more than 15% of entering class; international applicants considered.
University of Georgia	Up to 10 positions.
University of Illinois	20–30 positions.
Iowa State University	Up to 22 positions, plus unfilled contract positions; international applicants considered.
Kansas State University	50% of class; international applicants considered.
Louisiana State University	Up to 22 positions.
Michigan State University	20–25% of entering class; international applicants considered.
University of Minnesota	Not more than 40% of entering class.
Mississippi State University	35–40 positions.
University of Missouri	Minimum 16 positions.
North Carolina State University	Up to 14 positions.
Ohio State University	Up to 38 positions.

Oklahoma State University	Up to 20 positions; U.S. citizens and permanent residents only.
Oregon State University	Up to 8 positions.
University of Pennsylvania	50 positions; international applicants considered.
Purdue University	20 positions; international applicants considered.
University of Tennessee	20 positions.
Texas A & M University	Up to 10 positions.
Tufts University	Up to 40 positions; international applicants considered.
Tuskegee University	Up to 5 positions; international applicants considered.
Virginia-Maryland Regional College of Veterinary Medicine	Up to 10 positions.
Washington State University	Limited number of positions.
Western University of Health Sciences	Up to 100 positions for out-of-state applicants and up to 8 international positions.
University of Wisconsin	Up to 20 positions.

International

University of Edinburgh	Up to 25 positions available for international applicants.
University of Glasgow	24 positions for international applicants.
University of Guelph	5 positions for international applicants.
Massey University	24 positions for international applicants.
University of Prince Edward Island	Up to 24 positions for international applicants.

LISTING OF CONTRACTING STATES AND PROVINCES

Six Canadian provinces and 19 states in the United States have a veterinary school contract with one or more schools to provide access to veterinary medical education for their residents. The state or province, working through the contracting agency, usually agrees to pay a fee to help cover the cost of education for a certain number of places in each entering class. Residents from the contract states then compete with each other for those positions.

Some states contract with more than one school. For example, Arkansas contracts with 5 veterinary schools, and North Dakota has contracts with 6 schools. Connecticut, Rhode Island, Vermont, Nebraska, and the District of Columbia presently have no contracts, so all candidates from these places apply as nonresidents to veterinary schools of their choice.

The educational agreements between contracting agencies and veterinary schools differ. Under some contract arrangements, students pay in-state tuition; in others, they pay nonresident tuition. Some contract states require students to repay all or part of the subsidy that the state provided; others require veterinary graduates to return to practice in the state for a period of time. Applicants should be aware of their obligation to the state before agreeing to participate in a contract program.

Following is a list of states and provinces that have educational agreements with schools of veterinary medicine.

UNITED STATES

Arizona
Contracts through WICHE* with University of California, Colorado State University, Oregon State University, and Washington State University.

Arkansas
Contracts in past with Louisiana State University, University of Missouri, and Oklahoma State University. Contracts not all completed at time of printing; may be some changes.

Delaware
Contracts with Oklahoma State University and the University of Georgia.

* WICHE = Western Interstate Commission for Higher Education (offices in Boulder, Colorado)

Georgia
Contracts with Tuskegee University, in addition to having a school in the state.

Hawaii
Contracts through WICHE* with University of California, Colorado State University, Oregon State University, and Washington State University.

Idaho
Contracts with Washington State University.

Kentucky
Contracts with Auburn University and Tuskegee University.

Maine
Contracts with Tufts University.

Montana
Contracts through WICHE* with University of California, Colorado State University, Oregon State University, and Washington State University.

Nevada
Contracts through WICHE* with University of California, Colorado State University, Oregon State University, and Washington State University.

New Hampshire
Contracts with Cornell University and Tufts University.

New Jersey
Contracts with Cornell University, University of Illinois, Iowa State University, University of Pennsylvania, Oklahoma State University, Tufts University, and Tuskegee University.

New Mexico
Contracts through WICHE* with University of California, Colorado State University, Oregon State University, and Washington State University.

North Dakota
Contracts with Iowa State University and the University of Minnesota. Contracts through WICHE* with the University of California, Colorado State University, Oregon State University, and Washington State University.

* WICHE = Western Interstate Commission for Higher Education (offices in Boulder, Colorado)

13

Puerto Rico
Cooperative agreement with
University of Wisconsin.

South Carolina
Contracts with University of Georgia,
Mississippi State University,
and Tuskegee University.

South Dakota
Reciprocity with University of
Minnesota. Contracts with Iowa
State University.

Utah
Contracts through WICHE* with
University of California, Colorado
State University, Oregon State
University, and Washington State
University.

West Virginia
Contracts with University of
Georgia, Ohio State University, and
Tuskegee University.

Wyoming
Contracts through WICHE* with
the University of California,
Colorado State University, Oregon
State University, and Washington
State University.

CANADA

Alberta
Contracts with University of
Saskatchewan.

British Columbia
Contracts with University of
Saskatchewan.

Manitoba
Reciprocity with University of
Minnesota. Contracts with
University of Saskatchewan.

New Brunswick
Contracts with Atlantic Veterinary
College at the University of Prince
Edward Island and Université de
Montréal.

Newfoundland
Contracts with Atlantic Veterinary
College at the University of Prince
Edward Island.

Nova Scotia
Contracts with Atlantic Veterinary
College at the University of Prince
Edward Island.

* WICHE = Western Interstate Commission for Higher Education (offices in Boulder, Colorado)

PROGRAMS FOR MULTICULTURAL OR DISADVANTAGED STUDENTS

The Association of American Veterinary Medical Colleges affirms the value of diversity within the veterinary medical profession. The membership is committed to incorporating that belief into their actions by advocating the recruitment and retention of underrepresented persons as students and faculty and ultimately fostering their success in the profession of veterinary medicine. The Association believes that through these actions society and the profession will be well served.

Many schools have programs designed to facilitate entry into, and retention by, veterinary programs nationwide. These programs are directed at several levels, from high-school students to the student who has already been accepted by a veterinary college. Most of these programs will accept students from every state, regardless of the school(s) to which an individual might eventually apply or attend.

Following is an alphabetical list of schools by state and a short explanation of their programs:

University of California
Program: Summer Enrichment Program

Description: a 6-week summer program. The purpose of this program is to increase the academic preparedness of disadvantaged students through science-based learning skills development, clinical education, individual advising, and student development.

Eligibility: Educationally and/or economically disadvantaged. Must have completed at least one year of college with a minimum science GPA of 2.50 and demonstrated interest in veterinary medicine.

Program dates: July–August.

Contact: Office of the Dean–Student Programs, School of Veterinary Medicine, University of California, One Shields Avenue, Davis CA 95616; telephone: (530) 752-1383.

Sponsorship: School of Veterinary Medicine, University of California-Davis.

Colorado State University
Program: Vet Prep

Description: a one-year academic program that serves as a bridge to the professional veterinary medical program for disadvantaged (cultural, social, economic) applicants who ranked high but were denied admission during the current admissions process. Limited to 7 students who upon successful completion are guaranteed admission to the veterinary program.

Eligibility: disadvantaged students.

Contact: College of Veterinary Medicine and Biomedical Sciences, W102 Anatomy, Colorado State University, Fort Collins CO 80523; telephone: (970) 491-7053; email: DVMAdmissions@colostate.edu.

Sponsorship: College of Veterinary Medicine and Biomedical Sciences, Colorado State University.

Program: Vet Start

Description: a 7-year undergraduate and professional program for students who come to Colorado State from high school. Undergraduate and professional program scholarships are provided, and admission to the professional veterinary medical program is guaranteed upon successful completion of the undergraduate requirements. Mentoring, support services, and summer jobs are available to participants.

Eligibility: students who have a disadvantaged background (economic, cultural, or social) will be given special consideration. Students must be high-school graduates with fewer than 15 semester credits of college coursework. Selection is competitive. There are 5 positions per year for incoming freshman undergraduate students.

Program dates: begins fall semester; applications available online early January; application deadline March 1.

Contact: College of Veterinary Medicine and Biomedical Sciences, W102 Anatomy, Colorado State University, Fort Collins CO 80523; telephone: (970) 491-7051; email: PreVetAdviser@colostate.edu.

Sponsorship: College of Veterinary Medicine and Biomedical Sciences, Colorado State University.

Cornell University

Program: State University of New York Graduate Underrepresented Minority Fellowships

Description: all matriculating underrepresented minorities are eligible (not restricted by state residency). Minority fellowships include full tuition or tuition reduction.

Contact: Director of Financial Aid, College of Veterinary Medicine, S2-009 Schurman Hall, Cornell University, Ithaca NY 14853-6401; telephone (607) 253-3766; www.vet.cornell.edu/public/financialaid/.

Program: Regents Professional Opportunities Scholarships

Description: a financial assistance program for New York residents who are underrepresented minorities. Must agree to work in New York for a time after graduation.

Contact: Director of Financial Aid, College of Veterinary Medicine, S2-009

Schurman Hall, Cornell University, Ithaca NY 14853-6401; telephone (607) 253-3766; www.vet.cornell.edu/public/financialaid/.

Michigan State University

Program: Vetward Bound Program

Description: Vetward Bound offers 3 levels of programming, each with its own eligibility requirements. The program provides a review of basic science content, research and/or clinical experience, preparation for the GRE and MCAT, veterinary experience, food and fiber animal experience, study strategy development, and field experiences. Placement in a specific level is determined by program staff and is based on educational background.

Eligibility: multicultural and/or educationally/economically disadvantaged first-year students through prematriculants into the professional degree program.

Program dates: June–July.

Contact: Vetward Bound Coordinator, College of Veterinary Medicine, A-135 East Fee Hall, Michigan State University, East Lansing MI 48824-1316; telephone: (517) 355-6521; email: vetbound@cvm.msu.edu.

Mississippi State University

Program: Board of Trustees of State Institutions of Higher Learning Veterinary Medicine Minority Loan/Scholarship Program

Description: a financial assistance program for Mississippi residents who are underrepresented minorities. Must agree to work in Mississippi for at least 3 years following graduation.

Contact: Director of Student Financial Aid, Mississippi Institutions of Higher Learning, 3825 Ridgewood Road, Jackson MS 39211-6453; telephone: (601) 982-6570.

North Carolina State University

Program: UNC Campus Scholarship Program—Graduate Student Component

Description: UNC General Administration funds this program. Eligibility is limited to new or continuing full-time doctoral students who have financial need and who are residents of North Carolina as of the beginning of the award period (as determined under the *Manual to Assist the Public Higher Education Institutions of N.C. in the Matter of Student Resident Classification for Tuition Purposes*). Individuals who have been accepted to a master's degree program in a department offering the doctoral degree and who intend, and will be eligible, to pursue doctoral studies at NC State after completion of the requirements for the master's degree are also eligible. The program provides up to $4,000 annually for North Carolina residents.

Contact: Director of Diversity Affairs, College of Veterinary Medicine, North Carolina State University, 4700 Hillsborough Street, Box 8401, Raleigh, NC 27606; telephone: (919) 513-6262; website: www.cvm.ncsu.edu.

Program: Diversity Graduate Assistant Grant

Description: Funded by the North Carolina State University Graduate School, recipients must be full-time, new or continuing students pursuing master's and doctoral degrees at North Carolina State University. The program provides up to $4,000 annually. Both resident and nonresident students are eligible to apply.

Contact: Director of Diversity Affairs, College of Veterinary Medicine, North Carolina State University, 4700 Hillsborough Street, Box 8401, Raleigh, NC 27606; telephone: (919) 513-6262; website: www.cvm.ncsu.edu.

Note: North Carolina residents are encouraged to apply for both programs. However, the annual maximum award for these grant programs is a combined $4,000. The grant is awarded on an annual basis. Awardees must reapply each year.

Ohio State University

Program: Young Scholars Program

Description: this summer program is offered to seventh- through eleventh-grade students from Ohio. It provides hands-on science activities, academic enrichment exercises, and career exploration opportunities.

Eligibility: disadvantaged students recommended by their faculty.

Program dates: June to August each summer.

Sponsorship: the State of Ohio and The Ohio State University.

Program: Summer Research Opportunity Program

Description: this program is designed to promote the migration of minority undergraduate students into graduate research educational programs by providing them with summer research experiences. The student is provided with his or her individualized research problem by a faculty mentor and expected to carry that research through to publication.

Eligibility: the student must have completed 2 years of college work and have achieved at least a 2.50 cumulative GPA. The student must be an underrepresented minority or economically disadvantaged.

Contact: Graduate School, The Ohio State University, 230 North Oval Mall, Columbus OH 43210.

Sponsorship: the Big Ten Consortium for Institutional Studies.

University of Tennessee

Program: Program for African-American High-School Students

Description: provides students with an opportunity to work with veterinarians in their hometowns for 8 weeks during the summer. During 2 weeks, students will be guests of the College of Veterinary Medicine on the campus of The University of Tennessee, Knoxville.

Eligibility: African-American sophomores, juniors, or seniors who are residents of Tennessee and enrolled in a Tennessee high school. Applicants must have an interest in veterinary medicine as a potential career. Preference will be given to seniors. Students receive a stipend for satisfactory performance in the program.

Program dates: summer.

Contact: Associate Dean, The University of Tennessee, College of Veterinary Medicine, 2407 River Drive, Room A102, Knoxville TN 37996-4550.

Tuskegee University

Program: Health Careers Opportunity Program

Description: this 8-week preadmission activity is designed to facilitate the entry of "at risk" students and provide the skills necessary for successful transition to the professional school.

Eligibility: participation is targeted to minority and disadvantaged students who have completed at least 3 years of college and all preveterinary prerequisites. Participation is restricted to persons who have applied to the DVM program in the College of Veterinary Medicine, Nursing, and Allied Health and who have been recommended by the Veterinary Admissions Committee for evaluation to the program.

Program dates: summer before matriculation.

Contact: Assistant Dean, College of Veterinary Medicine, Nursing, and Allied Health, Tuskegee University, Tuskegee, AL 36088.

Sponsorship: this program is sponsored by a grant from the U.S. Department of Health and Human Services.

Program: Veterinary Science Training, Education and Preparation Institutes for Minority Students (Vet-Step I and II)

Description: Consists of 2 one-week programs designed to encourage high-achieving minority students to consider veterinary medicine as a career choice. The program offers students progressive learning experiences in reading comprehension, note-taking, medical vocabulary, etc.

Eligibility: Vet-Step I accepts 30 students from grades 9 and 10; Vet-Step II accepts students from Vet-Step I and from grade 12. Minority high-school honor students interested in the biomedical sciences are eligible to apply.

Program dates: Vet-Step I—June; Vet-Step II—July.

Contact: Coordinator, Vet-Step Program, College of Veterinary Medicine, Nursing, and Allied Health, Tuskegee University, Tuskegee AL 36088, (334) 727-8309.
Sponsorship: U.S. Department of Health and Human Services.

Virginia-Maryland Regional College of Veterinary Medicine
Program: Multicultural Academic Opportunities Program—Blacksburg
Description: a 10-week program providing opportunities to conduct scientific research; participate in clinical rotations within the veterinary teaching hospital; improve leadership, public speaking, and self-marketing skills; attend GRE preparatory classes; and learn about admission into graduate/ professional school.
Contact: Admissions Office at Blacksburg campus.

Program: Summer Research Apprenticeship Program—College Park
Description: a summer research program providing research experience to veterinary and preveterinary students from diverse backgrounds, including economic hardship and underrepresented racial/ethnic groups. Projects may include assisting in the planning, preparation, and data collection for controlled experiments, clinical trials, or epidemiological investigations; researching disease processes; and performing literature searches.
Contact: Admissions Office at College Park campus.
Scholarship Opportunities: a limited number of scholarships are available to assist minority DVM students.

Washington State University
Program: Short-Term Research Training Program for Veterinary Students
Description: a 3-month summer program designed to promote interest in research by veterinary students. Emphasis is on a hands-on research project supervised by a faculty member with a research program. Stipends are provided.
Eligibility: Washington-Idaho program veterinary students or ethnic minority veterinary students from other U.S. colleges of veterinary medicine.
Program dates: 3 months in the summer dependent upon the summer vacation of the College of Veterinary Medicine in which the veterinary student is enrolled.
Contact: Department of Veterinary Microbiology and Pathology, Washington State University, Pullman WA 99164-7040.
Sponsorship: The National Center for Research Resources.

University of Wisconsin

Program: Pre-College Enrollment Opportunity Program for Learning Excellence (PEOPLE)

Description: this program began in the summer of 1999 as a partnership between the Milwaukee Public Schools and the UW-Madison with a group of students who had just completed the ninth grade. New classes will be added each year, expanding to Madison area schools. The program is designed with a precollege track and a bridge program to undergraduate work and continues through a student's undergraduate career at University of Wisconsin-Madison. The main purposes are to promote academic preparation, increase enrollment in postsecondary institutions, and improve retention and graduation rates of minority and disadvantaged students.

Eligibility: students of one or more of the following ethnic heritages: African American, American Indian, Asian American, Hispanic/Latino. Other eligibility factors include economic disadvantage and current enrollment in or commitment to a college preparatory curriculum track.

Program dates: June–July summer residential programs and year-round nonresidential
programs.

Contact: Assistant Vice Chancellor, 117 Bascom Hall, University of Wisconsin- Madison, Madison, WI 53706; or Associate Director, University of Wisconsin- Madison Undergraduate Admissions, Armory and Gymnasium, 716 Langdon Street, Madison, WI 53706.

Program: University of Wisconsin-Madison NASA Sharp Plus Program

Description: an 8-week residential precollege program designed to increase the participation and success rates of students from minority groups that are historically underrepresented in mathematics and sciences. Students are matched with mentors (professors and research scientists) who are currently engaged in scientific research at the university or in an industrial setting.

Eligibility: rising high-school juniors or seniors who are U.S. citizens or nationals, at least 16 years of age, and have completed at least the tenth grade by the start of the program; have completed at least one semester of algebra and geometry and at least one year of biology, chemistry, or physics with a grade of B or better in each of these courses; speak and write English at a level that does not require significant assistance; and are committed to full participation throughout the 8-week program.

Program dates: June–August.

Contact: Assistant Vice Chancellor, Room 117 Bascom Hall, University of Wisconsin-Madison, Madison, WI 53706; or Program Coordinator, University of Wisconsin-Madison Medical School, 1140C Medical Science Center, Madison, WI 53706

Sponsorship: Quality Education for Minorities and NASA.

Scholarships: the School of Veterinary Medicine has scholarships and other support funding available for students. A portion of those funds come from private donors earmarked specifically for underrepresented groups and individuals who have experienced long-term disadvantages.

FINANCIAL AID INFORMATION

Financing your veterinary medical education requires careful planning, good money management skills, and a willingness to make short-term sacrifices to achieve long-range goals.

Many of you will apply for and receive some type of financial assistance during your undergraduate education. This will help you become somewhat familiar with the process, and to know that the rules and regulations governing programs can and do change periodically.

As a professional student, you will be entering a partnership with the financial aid office, which will require you to complete the appropriate financial aid forms accurately, meet required deadlines, and submit any additional information that may be requested. In return, the financial aid office will determine your aid eligibility and make awards based on the available programs. Your financial aid eligibility takes into account the cost of your education minus any other available resources. Amounts of assistance and the school policies for awarding assistance vary from one veterinary medical school to another and from year to year.

Any questions or concerns that you may have about this topic need to be directed to each of the appropriate financial aid offices to ensure that you receive accurate information and guidance.

Financing Your Veterinary Medical Education

Your education is one of the biggest investments you will make in your lifetime, and one of your most important goals should be to maximize the return on all of your investments. To reach this goal, you must take an active role in managing your financial resources. You need to understand and implement good financial practices. To get you started, here are some good financial habits you should adopt:

- Do not use credit cards to extend your lifestyle. Deciding not to use credit cards except in emergencies is one of the most important decisions you can make, and one that will reduce your stress while you are pursuing your education.

- Budget your money just as carefully as you budget your time. Contact a financial aid administrator to help you set up a budget that will be easy to follow.

- Distinguish between wants and needs. Before you make any purchase, you should ask yourself, "Do I need this, or do I want it?"

- Be a well-informed borrower. If you have not previously taken an active role in understanding the differences between various student loan programs, now is the time to do it. You need to know these differences in order to avoid high-interest loans and to borrow wisely.

- Borrow the minimum amount necessary in order to maximize the return on your educational investment.

- Be thrifty. Live as cheaply as you can. Remember, you are a student. You'll enjoy a more comfortable lifestyle once you are a DVM.

- Pay any interest that accrues on student loans if you can afford to do so, rather than let the interest accrue and capitalize. Any amount you pay while you're a student will save you money once you enter repayment.

What is the most important piece of advice for making the most of your educational investment? Don't live the lifestyle of a DVM until you have completed your education. Get in the habit of being thrifty. If you live like a DVM while you are in school, you may have to live like a student when you are a DVM.

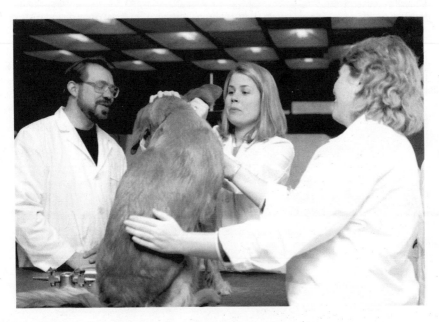

University of Minnesota faculty and student examine a dog.

Federal Loan Programs

	Subsidized Stafford Loan	Unsubsidized Stafford Loan
Lender	Financial or credit institution or eligible school	Financial or credit institution or eligible school
Financial Need	Yes	No
Citizenship Requirement	U.S. Citizen, U.S. National or U.S. Permanent Resident	U.S. Citizen, U.S. National or U.S. Permanent Resident
Borrowing Limits	$8,500/year; $65,500 aggregate undergraduate and graduate	Cost of attendance minus other aid; $189,125 aggregate undergraduate and graduate, less the Subsidized Stafford Loan Total
Interest Rate	Variable; capped at 8.25%	Variable; capped at 8.25%
Interest Accrues School	No	Yes
Deferments	No	Yes
Grace Period	No	Yes

Perkins Loan	Health Professions Student Loan	Loan for Disadvantaged Students
Veterinary Medicine Financial Aid Office	Veterinary Medicine Financial Aid Office	Veterinary Medicine Financial Aid Office
Yes	Yes	Yes
U.S. Citizen, U.S. National or U.S. Permanent Resident	U.S. Citizen, U.S. National or U.S. Permanent Resident	U.S. Citizen, U.S. National or U.S. Permanent Resident
$6,000/year; $40,000 aggregate undergraduate and graduate	Cost of attendance at participating school	Cost of attendance at participating school
5%	5%	5%
No	No	No
No	No	No
No	No	No

INFORMATION ABOUT STANDARDIZED TESTS

Most veterinary medical colleges require one or more standardized tests: the Medical College Admission Test (MCAT) or Graduate Record Examination (GRE®). For further information regarding test dates and registration procedures, contact the testing agencies listed below:

GRE Graduate Record Examination
P.O. Box 6000
Princeton NJ 08541-6000
(609) 771-7670 (Princeton, N.J.)
also: (510) 654-1200 (Oakland, Calif.)
www.gre.org
Individual school codes: see GRE booklet

MCAT Medical College Admission Test
MCAT Program Office
P.O. Box 4056
Iowa City IA 52243-4056
(319) 337-1357
www.aamc.org/students/mcat/

TOEFL Test of English as a Foreign Language
TOEFL/TSE Services
P.O. Box 6151
Princeton NJ 08541-6151
(609) 771-7100
www.toefl.org

VETERINARY MEDICAL COLLEGE APPLICATION SERVICE (VMCAS)

The Veterinary Medical College Application Service is a centralized application service sponsored by the Association of American Veterinary Medical Colleges. Applicants use VMCAS to apply to most of the AVMA accredited colleges in the United States and abroad.

VMCAS collects, processes, and ships application materials to veterinary colleges designated by the applicant, and responds to applicant inquiries about the application process. This service is the data collection, processing, and distribution component of the admission process for colleges participating in VMCAS. VMCAS, however, does not take part in the admissions selection process.

Twenty-five (25) of the twenty-eight (28) U.S. veterinary institutions participate in VMCAS, along with two (2) Canadian and (2) Scottish veterinary institutions. Application material deadlines, prerequisite courses, and other aspects of the admissions process differ from school to school. Applicants are responsible for being informed of all instructions provided by VMCAS and the associated member colleges. Questions about using VMCAS should be directed to the VMCAS Student & Advisor Hotline.

> VMCAS
> 1101 Vermont Ave NW
> Suite 301
> Washington, DC 20005
> Telephone (202) 682-0750
> Toll-Free Student & Advisor Hotline (877) 862-2740
> Fax (202) 682-1122
> vmcas@aavmc.org
> http://www.aavmc.org

VETERINARY MEDICAL SCHOOLS IN THE UNITED STATES

Auburn University

Office for Academic Affairs
Auburn University
College of Veterinary Medicine
217 Goodwin Student Center
Auburn University AL 36849-5536
Telephone: (334) 844-2685
Email: admiss@vetmed.auburn.edu
www.vetmed.auburn.edu

The College of Veterinary Medicine at Auburn University is located in south central Alabama off Interstate 85 between Montgomery and Atlanta. The university is known for its friendly small-campus atmosphere despite having more than 23,000 students.

Veterinary medicine began as a department at Auburn in 1892 and became a college in 1907. Today it is situated on 280 acres one mile from the main Auburn campus. In addition, the college has a 700-acre research farm five miles from its campus. The college is fully accredited by the American Veterinary Medical Association.

Application Information

For specific application information (availability, deadlines, fees, and VMCAS participation), please refer to the contact information listed above.

Residency implications: priority is given to Alabama residents. Auburn contracts with Kentucky for 34 positions. Up to 10 nonresident students are accepted.

Prerequisites for Admission

Course requirements and semester hours

Written composition#	6
* Literature#	3
Fine Arts#	3
Humanities/fine arts elective#	6
* History#	3
Social/behavioral science electives#	9

Mathematics—precalculus with trigonometry#	3
Biology I with lab	4
Biology II with lab	4
Fundamentals of chemistry with lab	8
**Organic chemistry with lab	6
**Physics	8
Biochemistry	3
Science electives (jr. [300] level or above)	6

* *Students must complete a 6-semester-hour sequence either in literature or in history.*

** *Organic chemistry and physics must have been taken within 6 calendar years.*

These requirements will be waived if the student has a bachelor's degree.

Required undergraduate GPA: a minimum grade point average of at least 2.50 on a 4.00 scale is required, with the minimum acceptable grade for required courses being C-minus. Applicants not classified as Alabama residents or contract students must have a minimum 3.00 GPA on a 4.00 scale. The mean grade point average of the most recent entering class was 3.46.

AP credit policy: must appear on official college transcripts and be equivalent to the appropriate college-level coursework.

Course completion deadline: prerequisite courses must be completed by June 15 prior to matriculation.

Standardized examinations: Graduate Record Examination (GRE®), general test, is required. The exam must have been taken within the previous 5 calendar years, and no later than November 30 of the year of application.

Additional requirements and considerations
    Animal/veterinary experience
    Recommendations (3 required)
     Academic advisor or faculty member
     Employer
     Veterinarian
    Extracurricular and community service activities
    Employment record
    Narrative statement of purpose
    Neatness of application
    Organic chemistry and physics courses must have been completed within the previous 6 calendar years

Summary of Admission Procedure

Timetable

Application deadline: October 2
Date interviews are held: February–March
Date acceptances mailed: March
School begins: August

Deposit (to hold place in class): none required.

Deferments: not considered.

Evaluation criteria
The 3-part admission procedure includes an objective evaluation of academic credentials, a subjective review of personal credentials, and a personal interview by invitation.

2005–2006 admissions summary

	Number of Applicants	Number of New Entrants
Resident	88	46
Contract*	102	34
Nonresident	613	13
Total:	803	93

Expenses for the 2005–2006 Academic Year

Tuition and fees

Resident	$10,178.00
Nonresident	
Contract*	$10,178.00
Other nonresident	$30,058.00

* For further information, see the listing of contracting states and provinces.

University of California

School of Veterinary Medicine
Office of the Dean—Student Programs
University of California
One Shields Avenue
Davis CA 95616
Telephone: (530) 752-1383
www.vetmed.ucdavis.edu

The University of California (UCD) Davis campus is one of 10 campuses of the University of California. It is the largest campus, with 5,200 acres. The Davis campus is set between the Coast Range to the west and the towering Sierra Nevada to the east in the heart of the Central Valley. The campus is close to California's state capital and the San Francisco Bay Area but cherishes its small-town culture and security. Davis is surround by open space, including some of the most productive agricultural land in the state. The terrain is flat, and 50 miles of bike paths crisscross the city. Davis has earned the title "City of Bicycles." Winters in Davis are generally mild. Summers are hot and dry, usually in the low 90s, although some days it can exceed 100 degrees. Spring and fall weather is some of the most pleasant in the state. UC Davis is an outstanding research and training institution with over 30,000 undergraduate, graduate and professional students. The Davis campus has three undergraduate colleges, graduate studies in all schools and colleges, and professional programs carried out in the schools of Law, Management, Medicine and Veterinary Medicine. The School of Veterinary Medicine is home of the Veterinary Medical Teaching Hospital, Veterinary Medicine and Teaching Research Center, California National Primate Research Center, California Animal Health and Food Safety Laboratory, UC Veterinary Medical Center-San Diego, Center for Companion Animal Health and Center for Equine Health. There are many other centers and innovative programs at UC Davis. The school is fully committed to recruiting students with diverse backgrounds.

Application Information

For specific application information (availability, deadlines, fees, and VMCAS participation), please refer to the contact information listed above.

Residency implications: priority is given to California residents. A small number of uniquely qualified nonresident applicants and WICHE applicants are accepted.

Prerequisites for Admission

Course requirements and quarter hours

General chemistry (with laboratory)	15
Organic chemistry (with laboratory)	6
Physics	6
Biology and zoology (1 laboratory requirement)	10
Systemic physiology*	5
Biochemistry* (bioenergetics and metabolism)	5
Genetics*	4
English composition and additional English	12
Humanities and social sciences	12
Statistics	4

* Upper-division courses equivalent to one semester or one quarter—labs not required. Note: equivalent courses may vary in units and may also require other prerequisites. All lower division courses are full year courses on the semester system.

Required undergraduate GPA: a minimum grade point average of 2.50 on a 4.00 scale is required for *both* the required sciences (listed above) and cumulative college coursework. Applicants admitted in fall 2005 had a mean cumulative GPA of 3.50.

AP credit policy: must appear on official college transcripts.

Course completion deadline: all prerequisite courses must be completed by the time a student plans to enroll. Half of the required courses must be completed at the time of application.

Standardized examinations: Graduate Record Examination (GRE®), general test, is required. The most recent acceptable GRE test date for applicants entering fall 2007 is October 2, 2006. Average GRE scores for the class admitted in 2005 are verbal 583, quantitative 702, and analytical writing 5.0.

Additional requirements and considerations

Veterinary/animal experience
Letters of evaluation (3)
Personal statement of motivation/career goals
Accuracy and neatness of application
Interview

Summary of Admission Procedure

Timetable
  Application deadline: October 2
  Date interviews are held: February to mid-March
  Date acceptances mailed: by April 1
  School begins: early September

Deposit (to hold place in class): none required.

Deferments: not considered.

Evaluation criteria	% weight
Grades	25
Test scores	25
Personal Statement/Essay/Animal and Veterinary Experience/References/Other	30
Interview	20

2004–2005 admissions summary

	Number of Applicants	Number of New Entrants
Resident	518	118
Contract*	77	0
Nonresident	299	4
Total:	894	122

Expenses for the 2005–2006 Academic Year

Tuition and fees

Resident	$21,702.00
Nonresident	$33,948.00
Contract student*	$33,948.00

* For further information, see the listing of contracting states and provinces. All nonresident and contract students are eligible for residency in California in one year.

Dual-Degree Programs

Combined DVM–graduate degree programs are available.
Visit our Veterinary Scientist Training Program information at
www.vetmed.ucdavis.edu/vstp.

Colorado State University

Office of the Dean
College of Veterinary Medicine and Biomedical Sciences
Colorado State University
1601 Campus Delivery
Fort Collins CO 80523-1601
Telephone: (970) 491-7052
Email: PreVetAdviser@colostate.edu (for general or preveterinary questions
   not answered on website)
   DVMAdmissions@colostate.edu (for those within one year of applica-
   tion to DVM)
www.cvmbs.colostate.edu

Colorado State University is located in Fort Collins, a city of about 126,000 in the eastern foothills of the Rocky Mountains about 65 miles north of Denver. Fort Collins has a pleasant climate and offers many cultural and recreational activities. Many of the state's ski areas lie within a short driving distance, making some of the best skiing in the world accessible. The nearby river canyons and mountain parks are beautiful scenic attractions and provide opportunities for hiking, fishing, photography, camping, and biking.

The College of Veterinary Medicine and Biomedical Sciences is composed of 5 major buildings that house the departments of biomedical sciences, environmental and radiological health sciences, and microbiology, immunology, and pathology. The James L. Voss Veterinary Teaching Hospital, one of the world's largest and best-equipped, houses the clinical sciences department. This department boasts a variety of unique units, including the internationally acclaimed Robert H. and Mary G. Flint Animal Cancer Center, Animal Population Health Institute, Integrated Livestock Management Program, and Gail Holmes Equine Orthopaedic Research Center. The hospital attracts a large caseload and offers students a wide variety of clinical experiences.

Application Information

For specific application information (availability, deadlines, fees, VMCAS participation, and supplemental application requirements), please refer to the contact information listed above.

Residency implications: positions are allocated as follows: Colorado 75, WICHE contracts 29–42 (Arizona, Hawaii, Montana, Nevada, New Mexico, North

Dakota, Utah, Wyoming), and nonsponsored 20–32. WICHE students must be certified by their states. Nonsponsored students can be from any state or country.

Prerequisites for Admission

Course requirements and semester hours

Laboratory associated with a biology course	1
Genetics	3
Laboratory associated with a chemistry course	1
Biochemistry	3
Physics (with laboratory)	4
Statistics/biostatistics	3
English composition	3
Social sciences and humanities	12
Electives	30

Required undergraduate GPA: No minimum requirement. The mean GPA for the 2005 matriculated class was 3.61 on a 4.00 scale.

AP credit policy: must appear on official college transcripts.

Course completion deadline: transcripts with final grades, including all required courses, must be received by July 15 prior to matriculation.

Standardized examinations: Graduate Record Examination (GRE®), general test, is required and must be taken within the last five years prior to application. Scores must be received by October 2, 2006. Mean GRE scores for the 2005 matriculated class were verbal 517, quantitative 637, analytical 4.55.

Additional requirements and considerations

Animal/veterinary/unique work experience
Recommendations (3) —must be submitted electronically
    Academic (academic advisor or college professor)
    Employer
    Veterinarian (at least 1 preferred)
Essay
Extracurricular and community service activities, leadership
Quality of academic program (course load, challenging curriculum, honors)
Contributions to diversity, extenuating circumstances

Summary of Admission Procedure

Timetable
    Application deadline: October 2
    Date interviews are held: early February
    School begins: late August

Deposit (to hold place in class): none required.

Deferments: not considered.

Evaluation criteria
    Grades, quality of academic program
    GRE® scores
    Animal/veterinary/other work experience
    Activities & achievements, community service
    Essay
    Letters of recommendation
    Interview (Colorado only)

2005–2006 admissions summary

	Number of Applicants	Number of New Entrants
Sponsored (Colorado)	246	75
Sponsored (WICHE)*	198	33
Nonsponsored	1,000	26
Total:	1,444	134

Estimated expenses for the 2006–2007 Academic Year

Tuition and fees (estimate, first 3 years)
    Sponsored (Colorado & WICHE) $12,366.00
    Nonsponsored $37,766.00

* For further information, see the listing of contracting states and provinces.

Dual-Degree Programs

Combined DVM–graduate degree programs are available (MBA/DVM, MSPH/DVM, & DVM/PhD).

Cornell University

Office of DVM Admissions
College of Veterinary Medicine
S2-009 Schurman Hall
Cornell University
Ithaca, NY 14853-6401
Telephone: (607) 253-3700
Email: vet_admissions@cornell.edu
www.vet.cornell.edu/admissions

Cornell is located in Ithaca, a college town of about 50,000 in the Finger Lakes region of upstate New York, a beautiful area of rolling hills, deep valleys, scenic gorges, and clear lakes. The university's 740-acre campus is bounded on two sides by gorges and waterfalls. Open countryside, state parks, and year-round opportunities for outdoor recreation, including excellent sailing, swimming, skiing, hiking, and other activities, are only minutes away.

Ithaca is one hour by air and a four-hour drive from New York City, and other major metropolitan areas are easily accessible. Direct commercial flights connect Ithaca with New York, Boston, Chicago, Pittsburgh, Philadelphia, and other cities.

The tradition of academic excellence, the cultural vigor of a distinguished university, and the magnificent setting create a stimulating environment for graduate study. The curriculum differs from other programs in that it is interdisciplinary, small group learning early in the program and focuses on the student as the primary force in learning.

Application Information

For specific application information (availability, deadlines, fees, and VMCAS participation), subscribe to our free newsletter sent via email. Pre-vets should subscribe at our website prior to applying and must be subscribed during the application cycle.

Residency implications: approximately 51 positions for New York State residents. Cornell contracts with New Hampshire and New Jersey.

Prerequisites for Admission

Course requirements and semester hours

English composition* or literature	6
Biology or zoology, full year with laboratory	6

* Three credits may be satisfied by a course in public speaking.

Physics, full year with laboratory	6
Inorganic (general) chemistry, full year with laboratory	6
Organic chemistry, full year with laboratory	6
Biochemistry	4
General microbiology, with laboratory	3
Non-prerequisite elective credits needed	53

All prerequisites must have a letter grade of C– or better.

Required undergraduate GPA: No specific GPA requirement, but the grade range of those admitted tends to be 3.00–4.00.

AP credit policy: not accepted for courses other than physics and inorganic chemistry.

Course completion deadline: all but 12 credits of the prerequisite coursework should be completed at the time of application, with at least one semester of any two-semester series underway. Any outstanding prerequisites must be completed by the end of the spring term prior to matriculation.

Standardized examinations: Graduate Record Examination (GRE®), general test, or the Medical College Admission Test (MCAT) is required. Test scores must be self-reported on your supplemental application. Test scores older than 5 years will not be accepted.

Additional requirements and considerations
> Animal/veterinary experience, knowledge, and motivation
> Recommendations/evaluations (3 required minimum)
>> Academic advisor
>> Animal-experience employers (1 required from each employer or experience)
>> Nonveterinary work-related experiences (optional)
> Essay
> Extracurricular and/or community service activities

Summary of Admission Procedure

Timetable
> VMCAS application deadline: October 2
> Supplemental application deadline: preferred Oct. 5
> extended Nov. 1
> Information sessions at the college: February
> Date acceptances mailed: January
> School begins: late August

Deposit (to hold place in class): $500.00.

Deferments: considered on an individual basis, and ordinarily granted for illness or other situations beyond the control of the applicant.

Evaluation criteria

The admission procedure consists of 2 phases: an objective evaluation of academic credentials and a subjective review of the overall application.

	% weight
Grades	25
Test scores	25
Animal/veterinary experience	20
References, essay, quality of academic program, nonacademic activities, and noncognitive attributes	30

2005–2006 admissions summary

	Number of Applicants	Number of New Entrants
Resident	241	47
Contract*	74	6
Nonresident	556	30
Total:	871	83

Expenses for the 2004–2005 Academic Year

Tuition and fees

Resident	$22,000.00
Nonresident	
Contract student*	$22,000.00
Other nonresident	$31,500.00

* For further information, see the listing of contracting states and provinces.

Dual-Degree Programs

Dual DVM–graduate degree programs are available. Our dual DVM/PhD program offers a $23,500 stipend and free tuition for 7 years.

Leadership Program

The Leadership Training Program targets gifted first-year veterinary medical students who are potential leaders in the profession. The major objective of the program is to acquaint students with veterinary medical career opportunities in academic institutions, government, and industry. The program also encourages networking among the participants. Fellowships are available.

University of Florida

Admissions Office
College of Veterinary Medicine
P.O. Box 100125
University of Florida
Gainesville FL 32610-0125
Telephone: (352) 392-4700, ext. 5300
Email: henryt@mail.vetmed.ufl.edu
www.vetmed.ufl.edu

The University of Florida is located in Gainesville, a college town of approximately 100,000 in north central Florida, midway between the Gulf of Mexico and the Atlantic Ocean. Changes in season are marked, but winters are mild and permit year-round participation in outdoor activities.

The university accommodates about 40,000+ students with programs in almost all disciplines. The College of Veterinary Medicine is a component of the Institute of Food and Agricultural Sciences (which also includes Agriculture and Forest Resources and Conservation). It is also one of 6 colleges affiliated with the Health Science Center (the other 5 are Dentistry, Health-related Professions, Medicine, Nursing, and Pharmacy).

The veterinary curriculum is a 9-semester program consisting of core curriculum and elective experiences. The core provides the body of knowledge and skills common to all veterinarians. The first 4 semesters concentrate primarily on basic medical sciences. Students are additionally introduced to physical diagnosis, radiology, and clinical problems during these years. The core also includes experience in each of the clinical areas. Elective areas of concentration permit students to investigate further the aspects of both basic and clinical sciences most relevant to their interests.

Application Information

For specific application information (availability, deadlines, fees, and VMCAS participation), please refer to the contact information listed above.

Residency implications: priority is given to Florida residents, and Florida has no contractual agreements. Nonresidents are considered in very limited numbers (not more than 15% of any entering class).

Prerequisites for Admission

Course requirements and semester hours

Biology (general, genetics, microbiology)	15
Chemistry (inorganic, organic, biochemistry)	19
Physics	8
Mathematics (calculus, statistics)	6
Animal Science (introduction to animal science, animal nutrition)	6
Humanities	9
Social sciences	6
English (2 courses in English composition)	6
Electives	at least 5

Required undergraduate GPA: a minimum GPA of 2.75 on a 4.00 scale. The class of 2009 had an overall mean science prerequisite GPA of 3.47.

AP credit policy: must appear on official college transcripts and be equivalent to the appropriate college-level coursework.

Course completion deadline: prerequisite courses must be completed by the end of the spring term prior to admission.

Standardized examinations: Graduate Record Examination (GRE®) is required. October 2006 is the most recent acceptable test date for applicants to the class of 2011. Mean score for the class of 2009 was 1201.

Additional requirements and considerations
    Animal/veterinary experience
    Recommendations/evaluations (3 required)
        Personal
        Veterinarian
        Academic advisor
    Honors and awards received
    Extracurricular activities
    Essay

Summary of Admission Procedure

Timetable
- Application deadline: October 2
- Date interviews are held: March
- Date acceptances mailed: April 1
- School begins: mid-August

Deposit (to hold place in class): none required.

Deferments: considered on an individual basis.

Evaluation criteria

The admission procedure consists of 3 parts: each applicant's file is reviewed; selected applicants are each interviewed for about 20 minutes by 3 faculty members; final selection of new class takes place.

2005–2006 admissions summary

	Number of Applicants	Number of New Entrants
Resident	272	69
Contract	N/A	N/A
Nonresident	498	19
Total:	770	88

Expenses for the 2005–2006 Academic Year

Tuition and fees

Resident	$13,735.00
Nonresident	$35,661.00

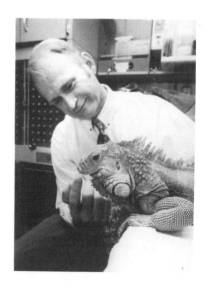

Not all of a veterinarian's patients are cuddly, especially for those specializing in wildlife and zoo medicine. Photo by Russ Lante, courtesy of University of Florida Health Science Center.

University of Georgia

Office for Academic Affairs
College of Veterinary Medicine
The University of Georgia
Athens GA 30602-7372
Telephone: (706) 542-5728
www.vet.uga.edu/admissions

The University of Georgia is located in Athens-Clarke County, with a population of over 100,000. Georgia's "Classic City" is a prospering community that reflects the charm of the Old South while growing in culture and industry (www. visitathensga.com). Athens is just over an hour away from the north Georgia mountains and the metropolitan area of Atlanta, and just over 5 hours away from the Atlantic coast.

In 1785, Georgia became the first state to grant a charter for a state-supported university. In 1801 the first students came to the newly formed frontier town of Athens. The University of Georgia has grown into an institution with 15 schools and colleges and more than 2,800 faculty members and 33,500 students.

Application Information

For specific application information (availability, deadlines, fees, and VMCAS participation), please refer to the contact information listed above.

Residency implications: Georgia retains up to 25 positions for contract students. Contracts are with Delaware (maximum 2), South Carolina (maximum 17), and West Virginia (maximum 6). The balance of those admitted are residents of Georgia or nonresident, noncontract applicants.

Prerequisites for Admission

Course requirements and semester hours

English	6
Humanities and social studies	14
General biology	8
Advanced biological science	8
Chemistry	
Inorganic	8
Organic	8
Physics	8
Biochemistry	3

Required undergraduate GPA: cumulative GPA of 3.00 or greater on a 4.00 scale *or* a combined score on the GRE® verbal and quantitative sections of 1200 or greater.

AP credit policy: must appear on official college transcripts and be equivalent to the appropriate college-level coursework.

Course completion deadline: prerequisite courses must be completed by the end of the spring term preceding entry.

Standardized examinations: Graduate Record Examination (GRE®), general test (including the analytical writing test), and the biology subject test must be completed within the 5 years immediately preceding the deadline for receipt of applications (October 2). Test scores must be received by December 31 after the October 2 application deadline.

Additional requirements and considerations
- Animal experience
- Background for veterinary medicine
- Recommendations/evaluations (3 required)
  - Academic advisor/faculty member (required for graduate students)
  - Employer
  - Veterinarian
- Essay

Summary of Admission Procedure

Timetable
- Application deadline: October 2
- Date acceptances mailed: late March
- School begins: late August

Deposit (to hold place in class): $100.00; $500.00 for nonresident, noncontract students.

Deferments: one-year deferments considered for reasons such as completing a degree or for health problems.

Evaluation criteria
The admissions procedure includes a file evaluation. There are no interviews.
  Program of study
  Animal/veterinary experience
  References
  Employment history
  Narrative statement
  Extracurricular activities

2004–2005 admissions summary

	Number of Applicants	Number Accepted
Resident	192	71
Contract*	94	24
Nonresident	280	1
Total:	566	96

Expenses for the 2004–2005 Academic Year

Tuition and fees (approximate)
Resident	$11,376.00
Nonresident	
Contract*	$11,376.00
Nonresident	$29,976.00

* For further information, see the listing of contracting states and provinces.

University of Illinois

Office of Academic and Student Affairs
College of Veterinary Medicine
University of Illinois at Urbana-Champaign
2271G Veterinary Medicine Basic Sciences Bldg.
2001 South Lincoln Avenue
Urbana IL 61802
Telephone: (217) 333-1192
Email: admissions@cvm.uiuc.edu
www.cvm.uiuc.edu

The University of Illinois is in Urbana-Champaign, a community of about 100,000 people located 140 miles south of Chicago. It is served by 4 airlines, 3 interstate highways, bus, and rail. The twin cities and university make a pleasant community with easy access to all areas and facilities. The university has about 35,000 students and more than 11,000 faculty and staff members. It is known for its high-quality academic programs and its exceptional resources and facilities. The university library has the largest collection of any public university and ranks third among all U.S. academic libraries. The university also has outstanding cultural and sports facilities and activities.

The College of Veterinary Medicine is located at the south edge of the campus in a large physical plant built in phases since 1971. In addition to approximately 400 students, the college has about 100 graduate students plus a full complement of residents and interns. There are more than 100 full-time faculty with research interests in a variety of biomedical sciences and clinical areas. This research activity allows a variety of interactions and employment for students. The college also offers students a stimulating core-elective curriculum to prepare for a career in almost any area of the profession.

Application Information

For specific application information (availability, deadlines, fees, and VMCAS participation), please refer to the contact information listed above.

Residency implications: priority is given to approximately 82 Illinois residents; approximately 30 nonresident positions.

Prerequisites for Admission

The academic requirements for application to the College of Veterinary Medicine can be met through one of two pathways: Plan A or Plan B. Those considering a career in veterinary medicine should have a good foundation in biological sciences and chemistry, including *biochemistry*, and should consider the specific courses listed in Plan A as a minimum knowledge base for success in the curriculum. In addition, a course or courses concerning livestock production and animal ethology are highly desirable for all students. Those seeking a career in veterinary medicine related to agriculture should consider additional background in nutrition, livestock management, and the economics of production by working toward a degree in animal science prior to admission to veterinary school.

Plan A

BS or BA degree in any major field of study from an accredited college or university including the following courses (equivalent in content to those required for students majoring in biological sciences):
  a. 8 semester hours of biological sciences with laboratories
  b. 16 semester hours of chemical sciences, including organic and bio-chemistry, with laboratories in inorganic and organic chemistry
  c. 8 semester hours of physics with laboratories

Plan B

Those applying without a bachelor's degree are required to present at least 60 semester hours from an accredited college or university, including 44 hours of science courses. The minimum course requirements under Plan B are:
  a. 8 semester hours of biological sciences with laboratories
  b. 16 semester hours of chemical sciences, including organic and bio-chemistry, with laboratories in inorganic and organic chemistry
  c. 8 semester hours of physics with laboratories
  d. 3 semester hours of English composition and an additional 3 hours of English composition and/or speech
  e. 12 semester hours of humanities and social sciences
  f. 12 semester hours of junior/senior-level science courses in addition to the requirements listed above

Required undergraduate GPA: a minimum cumulative GPA of 2.75 and a minimum science GPA of 2.75 on a 4.00 scale are required. The mean cumulative GPA for students invited to interview in 2004 was 3.50, mean science GPA was 3.36, and mean GRE® score was 68 (percentile).

AP credit policy: no AP credit given.

Standardized examinations: Graduate Record Examination (GRE®), general test, is required. Test must be taken by September 30 of the year of application, and scores may be no older than two years.

Additional requirements and considerations
> Animal veterinary knowledge, motivation, and experience
> Recommendations/evaluations
>> Animal- and veterinary-experience employer
>> Academic advisor
> Evidence of leadership, initiative, and responsibility
> Rigor of academic preparation

Summary of Admission Procedure

Timetable
> Application deadline: October 2
> Informational program and required interviews: early March
> Date acceptances mailed: mid-March
> School begins: late August

Deposit (to hold place in class): none required.

Deferments: considered on an individual basis.

Evaluation criteria
A 3-part admission procedure is used. An academic evaluation and a file evaluation of veterinary, animal experience and personal qualities are followed by a personal interview.

> Academic evaluation:
>> GRE® test scores
>> Science GPA
>> Cumulative GPA

> Nonacademic evaluation:
>> veterinary-related experience, animal-related experience, community involvement, leadership, citizenship, and letters of evaluation

> Interview

2003–2004 admissions summary

	Number of Applicants	Number of New Entrants
Resident	209	79
Nonresident	532	23
Total:	741	102

Expenses for the 2003–2004 Academic Year

Tuition and fees

Resident	$14,240.00
Nonresident	$34,704.00

Dual-Degree Programs

Combined DVM–graduate degree programs are available.

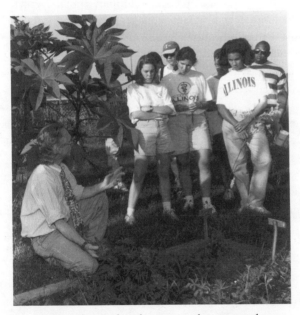

A professor of toxicology lectures in the poison plant garden at the University of Illinois College of Veterinary Medicine. Photo by Lil Morales, courtesy of the University of Illinois College of Veterinary Medicine.

Iowa State University

Office of Admissions
College of Veterinary Medicine
2270 Veterinary Medicine
Iowa State University
P.O. Box 3020
Ames IA 50010-3020
Telephone: (515) 294-5337
Toll free outside Iowa: (800) 262-3810
Email: cvmadmissions@iastate.edu
www.vetmed.iastate.edu

The Iowa State University College of Veterinary Medicine is located in the heart of one of the world's most intensive livestock-producing areas, which provides diverse food-animal clinical and diagnostic cases. A nearby metropolitan area and a regionally recognized referral veterinary hospital provide experience in companion-animal medicine and surgery. A strong basic science education during the first 2 years prepares veterinary students for a wide range of clinical experiences during the last 2 years. The College of Veterinary Medicine provides education in a wide variety of animal species and disciplines and allows fourth-year students to spend time with private practitioners, other colleges, research facilities, and in other educational experiences. Opportunities for research exist in the outstanding research programs in neurobiology, immunobiology, infectious diseases, and numerous other areas. The nearby National Animal Disease Center and the National Veterinary Services Laboratories provide additional research opportunities. The world's premier State Diagnostic Laboratory is part of the college and provides students with experience that is unmatched by any other veterinary college in the world. Graduates are highly sought after and can typically choose among 5 or 6 job offers. A career development and placement service is also provided.

Application Information

For specific application information (availability, deadlines, fees, and VMCAS participation), please refer to the contact information listed above.

Residency implications: priority is given to Iowa residents for approximately 60 positions. Iowa contracts on a year-to-year basis with Nebraska, New Jersey, North Dakota, and South Dakota. Remaining positions are available for residents of noncontract states or international students.

Prerequisites for Admission

Course requirements and semester hours

English composition[†]	6
General chemistry (1 year series w/lab)	7
Organic chemistry (1 year series w/lab)	7
Biochemistry	3
Physics (1 semester w/labs)	4
Biology (1 year series w/labs)	8
Genetics (Mendelian and molecular)	3
Mammalian anatomy and/or physiology	3
Oral communication (interpersonal, group or public speaking)	3
Arts, humanities, or social sciences	8
Electives	8

† English composition of one year or writing emphasis courses (may include business or technical writing).

Required undergraduate GPA: the minimum GPA required is 2.50 on a 4.00 scale. The most recent entering class had a mean GPA of 3.53.

AP credit policy: must be documented by original scores submitted to the university, and must meet the university's minimum requirement in the appropriate subject area. CLEP (College-Level Examination Program) credits accepted only for the arts, humanities, and social sciences.

Course completion deadline: It is preferred that prerequisite science courses be completed by the end of the fall term the year the applicant applies, and these must be completed with a C (2.0) or better to fulfill the requirement. However, up to 2 prerequisite science courses may be taken the spring term prior to matriculation, but the applicant must complete them with B (3.0) or better to fulfill the requirement. All other prerequisites must be completed by the end of the spring term prior to matriculation with a C (2.0) or better. Pending courses may not be completed the summer prior to matriculation. Pass–not pass grades are not acceptable.

Standardized examinations: Graduate Record Examination (GRE®), general test, is required.

Additional requirements and considerations
Recommendations (3 required). Academic advisors, veterinarians, and employers are suggested.

Summary of Admission Procedure

Timetable
  Application deadline: October 2
  Date acceptances mailed: Approximately February 15
  School begins: late August

Deposit (to hold place in class): $500.00.

Deferments: considered on a case-by-case basis.

Evaluation criteria
The admission procedure consists of a review of each candidate's application and qualifications:
  1. Academic factors include grades, test scores, and degrees earned.
  2. Nonacademic factors include essays, experience, recommendations, and personal development activities.
  3. Interviews were not conducted.

2004–2005 admissions summary

	Number of Applicants	Number of New Entrants
Resident	110	61
Contract*	110	36
Nonresident	331	23
Total:	551	120

Expenses for the 2006–2007 Academic Year

Tuition and fees

Resident	$13,860.00
Nonresident	
Contract*	varies by contract
Other nonresident	$34,197.00
Fees (approximate)	$800.00

* For further information, see the listing of contracting states and provinces.

Dual-Degree Programs

Combined DVM–graduate degree programs are available.

Kansas State University

Office of Student Admissions
College of Veterinary Medicine
101 Trotter Hall
Kansas State University
Manhattan KS 66506-5601
Telephone: (785) 532-5660
Fax: (785) 532-5884
Email: admit@vet.k-state.edu
www.vet.k-state.edu

Kansas State University in Manhattan, Kansas, is located 125 miles west of Kansas City near Interstate 70. With a population of about 68,000 including KSU, Manhattan is in an area surrounded by many historical points of interest in a rich agricultural area of north central Kansas. Recreational activities abound in Manhattan and the surrounding area with fishing, boating, camping, and hunting among the favorites. Sporting events, theater, concerts, and excellent parks contribute to the many activities available. Kansans enjoy the 4 seasons, each of which brings its own special activities and events.

Kansas State University is on a beautiful 664-acre campus. The College of Veterinary Medicine opened in 1905. It is located on 80 acres just north of the main campus in 3 connected buildings.

Application Information

For specific application information (availability, deadlines, fees, and VMCAS participation), please refer to the contact information listed above.

Residency implications: priority is given to Kansas residents; to be eligible to be in the Kansas pool of applicants, the applicant must be a Kansas resident for tuition purposes at the time of application. Kansas accepts about 60 nonresident students per year. International applicants are considered. Kansas has a contract for 2 students from North Dakota.

Prerequisites for Admission

Course Requirements and Semester Hours

Expository writing I and II	6
Public speaking	2
Chemistry I and II	8

General organic chemistry, with laboratory	5
General biochemistry, with laboratory	5
Physics I and II	8
Principles of biology or general zoology	4
Microbiology, with laboratory	4
Genetics	3
Social sciences and /or humanities	12
Electives	9

All science courses must have been taken within six years of the date of enrollment in the professional program.

Required undergraduate GPA: the required GPA to qualify for an interview is 2.80 on a 4.00 scale in both the prerequisite courses and the last 45 semester hours of undergraduate work. The most recent entering class had a mean prerequisite science GPA of 3.40.

AP credit policy: must appear on official college transcripts and be equivalent to the appropriate college-level coursework.

Course completion deadline: prerequisite courses must be completed by the end of the spring term of the year in which admission is sought.

Standardized examinations: Graduate Record Examination (GRE®), general test, scores are required by October 2.

Additional requirements and considerations
  Animal/veterinary work experience and knowledge
  Employment record
  3 evaluations required by nonfamily members, one a veterinarian. Other suggested references include academic or preprofessional advisor, professor, or other professional.

Summary of Admission Procedure

Timetable
  Application deadline: October 2
  Date interviews are held:
    Kansas residents: late December
    Nonresident: early January
    North Dakota: February

Date acceptances mailed: within 3 weeks after interview
School begins: mid-August

Deposit (to hold place in class): $100.00 for Kansas residents, $250.00 for non-resident students.

Deferments: may be considered by Admissions Committee for extraordinary circumstances.

Evaluation criteria
A 4-part admission procedure is used, including evaluation of science grades, evaluation of all 3 GRE® scores, assessment of the application and narrative, and a personal interview.

Prerequisite science GPA	30%
Test scores	40%
Interview score including:	30%

    References
    Animal/veterinary experience
    Leadership in college and community
    Autobiographical essay

2005–2006 admissions summary

	Number of Applicants	Number of New Entrants
Resident	119	45
Nonresident	445	61
North Dakota	16	2
Total:	580	108

* For further information, see the listing of contracting states and provinces.

Expenses for the 2005–2006 Academic Year

Tuition and fees (subject to change)

Resident	$12,362.00
Nonresident	$32,166.00

* For further information, see the listing of contracting states and provinces.

Dual-Degree Programs

Combined DVM–graduate degree programs are available.

Early Admission Program

The Veterinary Scholars Early Admission Program is designed for those students having a genuine desire to enter the veterinary profession who attend Kansas State University with an ACT score of 29 or greater or an equivalent SAT score and who complete a successful interview during the fall semester of their freshman undergraduate year.

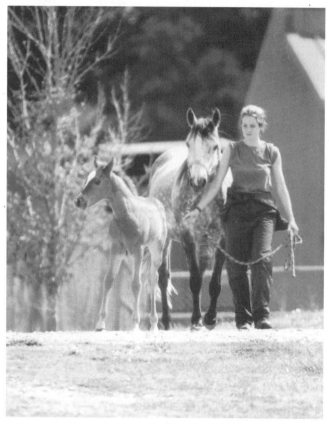

Veterinary students assist patients with rehabilitation schedules that include daily exercise. Photo courtesy of North Carolina State University College of Veterinary Medicine.

Louisiana State University

Office of Student and Academic Affairs
School of Veterinary Medicine
Louisiana State University
Baton Rouge LA 70803
Telephone: (225) 578-9537
Fax: (225) 578-9546
Email: cmiceli@vetmed.lsu.edu
www.vetmed.lsu.edu

The Louisiana State University campus is located in Baton Rouge, which has a population of more than 500,000 and is a major industrial city, a thriving port, and the state's capital. Since it is located on the Mississippi River, Baton Rouge was a target for domination by Spanish, French, and English settlers. The city bears the influence of all 3 cultures and offers a range of choices in everything from food to architectural design. Geographically, Baton Rouge is the center of south Louisiana's main cultural and recreational attractions. Equally distant from New Orleans and the fabled Cajun bayou country, there is an abundance of cultural and outdoor recreational activities. South Louisiana has a balmy climate that encourages lush vegetation and comfortable temperatures year round.

The campus encompasses more than 2,000 acres in the southern part of Baton Rouge and is bordered on the west by the Mississippi River. The Veterinary Medicine Building, occupied in 1978, houses the academic departments, the veterinary library, and the Veterinary Teaching Hospital and Clinics. The school is fully accredited by the American Veterinary Medical Association.

Application Information

For specific application information (availability, deadlines, fees, and VMCAS participation), please refer to the contact information listed above.

Residency implications: Louisiana contracts with Arkansas (9). Louisiana accepts up to 22 highly qualified nonresident applicants.

Prerequisites for Admission

Course requirements and semester hours

Biology	8
Microbiology	4
Physics	6
General chemistry	8
Organic chemistry	3
Biochemistry	3
English composition	6
Speech communication	3
Mathematics	5
Electives	20

Required undergraduate GPA: the minimum acceptable GPA for required coursework is 3.00 on a 4.00 scale. The mean GPA of the most recent entering class at the time of acceptance was 3.78.

AP credit policy: must appear on official college transcripts and be equivalent to the appropriate college-level coursework.

Course completion deadline: prerequisite courses must be completed by the end of the spring term preceding matriculation.

Standardized examinations: Graduate Record Examination (GRE®), general test, is required. The scores must be received by December 15. The average GRE combined verbal and quantitative score was 1140 for the class of 2008.

Additional requirements and considerations
  Animal/veterinary work experience
  Motivation, maturity, leadership skills
  Demonstrated communication skills
  Breadth of interests
  Entrepreneurial and business skills

Summary of Admission Procedure

Timetable
  Application deadline: October 3
  Supplemental application deadline: December 1
  Date interviews (Arkansas and Louisiana residents only) are held: February
  Date acceptances mailed: late March
  School begins: mid-August

Deposit (to hold place in class): $500.00 for nonresidents.

Deferments: considered.

Evaluation criteria

The approximate components of the evaluation scoring are:

   Objective evaluation:

GPA required courses	32%
GPA last 45 hours	20%
Test scores	18%

   Subjective evaluation:

Animal/veterinary experience, references (3 required, one by a veterinarian), essay	15%
Personal interview	10%
Committee evaluation	5%

2005–2006 admissions summary

	Number of Applicants	Number of New Entrants
Resident	135	54
Contract*	40	9
Nonresident	624	21
Total:	799	84

Expenses for the 2005–2006 Academic Year

Tuition and fees (estimated)

Resident	$11,856.00
Nonresident	
Contract*	$11,856.00
Other nonresident	$30,456.00

* For further information, see the listing of contracting states and provinces.

Michigan State University

Office of Admissions
College of Veterinary Medicine
F-104 Veterinary Medical Center
Michigan State University
East Lansing MI 48824-1316
Telephone: (517) 353-9793; fax: (517) 432-2391;
Helpline: (800) 496-4MSU (4678)
Email: admiss@cvm.msu.edu
www.cvm.msu.edu

Michigan State University's campus is bordered by the city of East Lansing, which offers sidewalk cafes, restaurants, shops, and convenient mass transit. The campus is traversed by the Red Cedar River and has many miles of bike paths and walkways. This park-like setting provides an ideal venue in which MSU's 43,000 students may enjoy outdoor concerts and plays, canoeing, and cross-country skiing. North of the river is the older part of campus. The ivy-covered buildings, some built before the Civil War and listed on the National Register of Historic Places, house 5 colleges, the student union, and 10 residence halls. South of the river are more recent additions to the campus, such as the Wharton Center for Performing Arts, the Jack Breslin Student Events Center, and several intramural sports facilities.

The college is a national leader in state-of-the-art technology and facilities. A lecture hall is equipped with a computer at each of the 116 work stations. These computers are part of a network that links all parts of the Veterinary Medical Center and allows instructors to receive immediate feedback on how well students understand the lecture material. The Veterinary Teaching Hospital has one of the largest caseloads in the country. Outstanding faculty are involved in teaching veterinary students, providing patient treatment and diagnostic services, and conducting veterinary research.

Application Information

For specific application information (availability, deadlines, fees, and VMCAS participation), please refer to the contact information listed above.

Residency implications: priority given to Michigan residents. Admission of non-resident and international applicants is limited. Michigan State University has no contractual agreements.

Prerequisites for Admission

Course requirements and semester hours

General education

English composition	3
Social and behavioral sciences	6
Humanities	6

Mathematics and biological and physical sciences

General inorganic chemistry (with laboratory)	3–5
Organic chemistry (with laboratory)	6–8
Biochemistry*	4
General biology (with laboratory)	6–9
College algebra and trigonometry	3–5
College physics (with laboratory)	8

* This should be an upper-division course in general biochemistry.

The CVM faculty have approved the following 4 courses to be added to the admissions requirements for applicants entering in fall 2007 (class of 2011):

Animal Nutrition	2
Genetics	3–4
Cell biology (upper division)	3–4
Microbiology (with laboratory)	3–4

Required undergraduate GPA: none; the mean cumulative GPA for the last entering class (fall 2004) was 3.53 on a 4.00 scale.

AP credit policy: no AP credit given.

Course completion deadline: prerequisite courses must be completed by the end of the summer session prior to matriculation.

Standardized examinations: Medical College Admission Test (MCAT) or the Graduate Record Examination (GRE®), general test, is required no later than October 3. For applicants to the class of 2010, the most recent acceptable MCAT test scores are those of the August 2004 exam. The average MCAT scores for the class entering in 2004 were: verbal 8, physical sciences 7, and biological sciences 8. For applicants to the class of 2010, the most recent acceptable GRE test scores are those of the September 30, 2005 exam. For the class entering in 2004, average GRE scores were: verbal 509 and quantitative 650. The Test of English as a Foreign Language (TOEFL) is required for applicants whose primary language is not English.

Additional requirements and considerations

Extracurricular and/or community service activities
Veterinary-related experience
Evaluations—3 required
Veterinarian (1)
Applicant's choice (2)
Academic advisor (required for graduate students)

Summary of Admission Procedure

Timetable

Application deadline: October 2
(It is strongly recommended that VMCAS application, electronic evaluation letters, tests, and transcripts be submitted by Sept. 15.)

Transcripts from all institutions attended must be submitted to MSU-CVM by October 2. Failure to meet this deadline will result in withdrawal of your application. International transcripts must be evaluated by World Education Services (WES).

Interviews are required for invited applicants (November–February)
Date acceptances mailed: early April
School begins: late August

Deposit (to hold place in class): $500.00 for residents; $1,000.00 for nonresidents.

Deferments: are rare.

Evaluation criteria
The 5-step admission process consists of an academic review and a nonacademic review, including an interview and a pre-interview extemporaneous composition.

2005–2006 admissions summary

	Number of Applicants	Number of New Entrants
Resident	211	79
Nonresident	633	29
International	39	
Total:	883	108

Expenses for the 2004–2005 Academic Year

Tuition and fees

Resident	$16,164.00
Nonresident	$33,764.00

Early Admission Program/Veterinary Scholars Admission Program

The Veterinary Scholars Admission Program has been established by the College of Veterinary Medicine in cooperation with the Honors College at Michigan State. This program provides an admission opportunity for students who wish to complete a bachelor's degree consisting of advanced, intellectually challenging, and scholarly studies in concert with their entry to the four-year professional veterinary medical degree program. Enrollment at MSU and membership in the Honors College are required to be eligible for this option. Further information may be obtained from the Pre-veterinary Advising Center at the address indicated on page 17. For information on Honors College membership, contact: Honors College, 103 Eustace Hall, Michigan State University, East Lansing, MI 48824; telephone (517) 355-2326; or visit their website at http://www.msu.edu/unit/honcoll/.

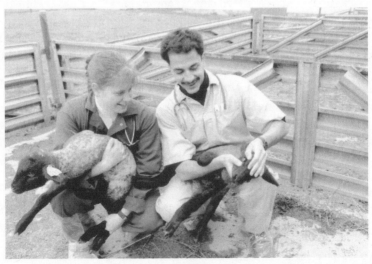

Students specializing in livestock veterinary medicine have many opportunities to gain practical skills. Photo courtesy of University of Minnesota College of Veterinary Medicine.

University of Minnesota

Office of Academic and Student Affairs
College of Veterinary Medicine
460 Veterinary Medical Center
1365 Gortner Avenue
University of Minnesota
St. Paul MN 55108
Telephone: (612) 624-4747
Email: dvminfo@umn.edu
www.cvm.umn.edu

The University of Minnesota's College of Veterinary Medicine is located on the 540-acre St. Paul campus. Students enjoy a small-campus atmosphere as well as the academic, cultural, social, and recreational opportunities of a major university and large metropolitan area. Cultural life includes world-renowned institutions and a rich local mix of theater, music, and arts organizations. The Twin Cities also house the state capital and the headquarters of many diverse major corporations. Minneapolis and St. Paul consistently rank near the top on quality-of-life and residential satisfaction ratings.

The College of Veterinary Medicine blends cornfields with biotechnology and cow barns with state-of-the-art diagnostic laboratories. The college provides contemporary facilities, including the Veterinary Medical Center, which is one of the most modern, well-equipped veterinary teaching hospitals in the country, and the Raptor Center, which in 1988 became the world's first facility designed specifically for birds of prey. The educational opportunities extend beyond the campus to include farms throughout Minnesota and around the world. Students are given opportunities to learn about the practice of contemporary veterinary medicine through externships, clinical rotations, and first-hand experiences with practitioners.

Application Information

For specific application information (availability, deadlines, fees, and VMCAS participation), please refer to the contact information listed above.

Residency implications: first priority is given to residents of Minnesota and residents of states/provinces with which a reciprocity agreement exists (North Dakota, South Dakota, Manitoba). Residents of other states are encouraged to apply. International applicants are only considered if their preveterinary courses have been completed at a U.S. college or university.

Prerequisites for Admission

Course requirements and quarter hours

Freshman English, communication	6–9
Mathematics	3–5
Chemistry (with laboratory)	
General inorganic	8–12
General organic*	5–10
Biology (with laboratory)	3–5
Zoology/animal biology (with laboratory)	3–5
Physics (with laboratory)	8–12
Biochemistry	3–5
Genetics	3–5
Microbiology (with laboratory)	3–5
Liberal education	12–18

* Two quarters with one laboratory or one semester with laboratory

A minimum of 4 courses from the following areas of study: anthropology, art, economics, geography, history, humanities, literature (including foreign language literature), music, political science, psychology, public speaking or small group (interpersonal) communication, social science, sociology, theater. No more than 2 courses can be from the same area of study.

Required undergraduate GPA: no minimum required. The class of 2009 had a mean GPA of 3.61 (on a 4.00 scale) for required courses and 3.70 for the last 60 quarter-hour or 45 semester-hour credits of coursework prior to admission.

AP credit policy: must appear on official college transcripts and be equivalent to the appropriate college-level coursework.

Course completion deadline: prerequisite courses must be completed by the end of the spring term (not later than June 15) of the academic year in which application is made.

Standardized examinations: Graduate Record Examination (GRE®), general test, is required and must be taken by October 2 with results received by October 31. The mean combined score for the verbal and quantitative sections of the GRE for the class entering in fall 2005 was 1170.

Summary of Admission Procedure

Timetable

Application deadline: October 2
Date acceptances mailed: mid-March
School begins: early September

Deposit (to hold place in class): $250.00.

Deferments: can be requested for special circumstances that warrant a 1-year delay in admission.

Evaluation criteria
  Objective measures of educational background
    Animal/veterinary knowledge, experience, and interest
    GPA in required courses
    GPA in recent courses
    Test scores
  Behavioral interviews
  Subjective measures of personal experience
    Employment record
    Extracurricular and/or community service activities
    Leadership abilities
    References
    Maturity/reliability

2004–2005 admissions summary

	Number of Applicants	Number of New Entrants
Resident*	194	55
Nonresident	557	35
Total:	751	90

The figures for new entrants include students taking delayed admission from the previous year.

*Includes residents of North and South Dakota and Manitoba.

Expenses for the 2006–2007 Academic Year

Tuition and fees (approximate)

Residents	$19,066.00
North Dakota residents	$31,550.00
Nonresidents	$35,802.00

Mississippi State University

Office of Student Affairs
College of Veterinary Medicine
P.O. Box 6100
Mississippi State University
Mississippi State MS 39762
Telephone: (662) 325-1278
Email: coats@cvm.msstate.edu
www.cvm.msstate.edu

Starkville is home to more than 16,000 MSU students and their Bulldogs. Starkville is located in northeast central Mississippi and has a population of 22,000. Being a land-grant university, MSU is green and beautifully landscaped. The university includes 9 farms scattered throughout the state. The College of Veterinary Medicine (the Wise Center) was completed in 1982. The college includes 620 rooms on 8 acres, or 360,000 square feet, under one roof.

The curriculum of the MSU-CVM is divided into 2 phases: Phase 1 (freshman and sophomore years) and Phase 2 (junior and senior years).

- Year 1 uses foundation courses to expose the student to important medical concepts and address multidisciplinary problems.

- Year 2 is devoted to the study of clinical diseases and abnormalities of various animal species. Surgery labs begin in the second year.

- Year 3 is comprised of clinical rotations in the College's Animal Health Center, and elective courses.

- Year 4 is largely experiential and offers the student the opportunity, once required courses have been scheduled, to select among approved experiences in advanced clinical rotations, elective courses, or externships.

The first 3 years of the curriculum are 9–10 months in length, while the fourth year is 12 months.

Application Information

For specific application information (availability, deadlines, fees, and VMCAS participation), please refer to the contact information listed above.

Residency implications: Mississippi accepts 35–40 nonresident students and has 5 contract positions with South Carolina.

Prerequisites for Admission

Course requirements and semester hours

English composition	6
Speech	3
Mathematics (college algebra or higher)*	6
Vertebrate zoology or anatomy with lab*	4
Microbiology with lab*	4
Immunology*	3
Genetics*	3
General chemistry with lab*	8
Organic chemistry with lab*	4
Biochemistry*	3
Physics with lab (may be trig-based)*	3
Nutrition (biochemically based, animal or human)	3–5
Humanities, fine arts, social and behavioral sciences	15

* Science and mathematics courses must be completed or updated within six calendar years prior to the anticipated date of enrollment.

Required undergraduate GPA: a minimum GPA of 3.0 on a 4.0 scale overall and in required math/science courses. Minimum GPA must be maintained throughout the application process. The class of 2009 has an average undergraduate GPA of 3.60.

AP credit policy: must appear on official college transcripts and be equivalent to the appropriate college-level coursework.

Course completion deadline: prerequisites must be completed by the end of the spring term prior to fall matriculation.

Standardized examinations: Graduate Record Exam (GRE®), general test, is required (no minimum score) and is due at the school by October 2.

Additional requirements and considerations

Evaluation of written application (including veterinary/research experience)

Supplemental application

Confidential evaluations

Interview (by invitation on a competitive basis)

Summary of Admission Procedure

Timetable

Application deadline: October 2
Date interviews are held: February
Date acceptances mailed: February
School begins: early August

Deposit (to hold place in class): $500.00.

Deferments: requests are considered on an individual basis.

Evaluation criteria

Grades
Quality of academic program
Test scores
Interview; animal/veterinary experience
References (3 required, one by a veterinarian)
Application (includes essay)

2005–2006 admissions summary

	Number of Applicants	Number of New Entrants
Resident	56	36
Nonresident	324	36
Total:	380	72

Expenses for the 2005–2006 Academic Year

Tuition and fees

Resident	$10,480.00
Nonresident	$31,843.00

Dual-Degree Programs

Combined DVM–graduate degree programs are available.

University of Missouri

Office of Academic Affairs
College of Veterinary Medicine
W203 Veterinary Medicine Building
University of Missouri-Columbia
Columbia MO 65211
Telephone: (573) 884-6435
Email: seayk@missouri.edu
www.missouri.edu

The University of Missouri-Columbia is located among rolling forested hills just north of the famous Lake of the Ozarks. Columbia is noted for its high quality of life and low cost of living and is consistently rated among the best cities to live in by *Money Magazine*. The city abounds with walking trails, 3,000 acres of state park lands, federal forests, and wildlife refuges. Columbia is located between Kansas City and St. Louis—cities that have major-league sports teams and other big-city recreational amenities. Columbia itself offers Big 12 Conference football, basketball, baseball, and other sports. It boasts a 65,000-seat stadium, several 18-hole golf courses, and other indoor and outdoor recreation facilities. Our location near a metropolitan area provides a strong primary and referral small animal case load. Columbia's proximity to rural central Missouri results in an exceptional food animal and equine case load.

MU, a major research university with 27,000 students, consists of 17 schools and colleges located on a 1,335-acre campus. The College of Veterinary Medicine is noted for its unique curriculum that gives students 2 years of undiluted clinical experience before graduation as opposed to the traditional 1–1½ years. Students benefit from exposure to specialty medical areas such as clinical cardiology, neurology, orthopedics, ophthalmology, and oncology. Students also gain experience with advanced equipment such as a linear accelerator for treatment of cancer, MRI, state-of-the-art ultrasonography, extensive endoscopy equipment, cold lasers, a surgery room C-arm for radiography during surgical procedures, and others. MU is unique in having a medical school, nursing school, school of health-related professions, state cancer research center, and department of animal science on the same campus, thus enhancing teaching, research, and clinical services.

Application Information

For specific application information (availability, deadlines, fees, and VMCAS participation), please refer to the contact information listed above.

Residency implications: first priority is given to Missouri residents; second priority is given to nonresidents. U.S. citizenship or permanent residency is required.

Prerequisites for Admission

Course requirements and semester hours

English or communication	6
College algebra or more advanced mathematics	3
Inorganic chemistry	8
Organic chemistry (with laboratory)	5
Physics	5
Biological science	10
Social sciences or humanities	10
Electives	10
Biochemistry	3

Required undergraduate GPA: a cumulative GPA of 2.50 or more on a 4.00 scale is required for Missouri residents. Nonresidents must have a cumulative GPA of 3.00 or more. The most recent entering class had a mean GPA of 3.57 at the time of acceptance.

AP credit policy: not accepted unless documented on University of Missouri transcript.

Course completion deadline: prerequisite courses must be completed by the end of the winter semester or spring quarter of the year of entry.

Standardized examinations: The Medical College Admission Test (MCAT) or the Graduate Record Examination (GRE®) general test is required. Test scores older than 3 years will not be accepted.

Additional requirements and considerations
Animal/veterinary experience
Recommendations/evaluations (3 required)
    Employer
    Academic advisors/faculty member
    Veterinarians
Extracurricular and/or community service activities
Essays
 Animal experience
 Explanation of choice of veterinary medicine as a profession
Employment history

Summary of Admission Procedure

Timetable

  VMCAS application deadline: October 2
  Direct application and supplemental application deadline: November 1
  Date interviews are held: February–March
  Date acceptances mailed: mid-April
  School begins: late August

Deposit (to hold place in class): $100.00 for residents; $250.00 for nonresidents.

Deferments: each is considered individually by the admissions committee.

Evaluation criteria
The admission process consists of a file review of all applicants and a personal interview of residents only.

	% weight
Grades	45
Test scores	5
Animal/veterinary experience	25
Interpersonal skills	15
Work ethics	5
Diversity	5

2005–2006 admissions summary

	Number of Applicants	Number of New Entrants
Resident	94	62
Nonresident	101	10
Total:	195	72

Expenses for the 2005–2006 Academic Year

Tuition and fees

Resident	$14,930.00
Nonresident	$28,620.00

Dual-Degree Programs

Combined DVM–graduate degree programs are available.

Early Admission Program

The Pre-veterinary Medicine and AgScholars Programs guarantee acceptance into the professional program upon satisfactory completion of the undergraduate requirements. Eligibility requires a high-school senior or University of Missouri freshman to have a composite ACT score of at least 30 and 27 respectively, or an equivalent SAT score. Eligible applicants will be interviewed, and a satisfactory score must be achieved to become a Scholar. Selected veterinary medical faculty will be assigned as mentors. Scholars receive priority consideration for part-time employment in the college. Further information may be obtained by contacting the Office of Academic Affairs at the address indicated on page 72.

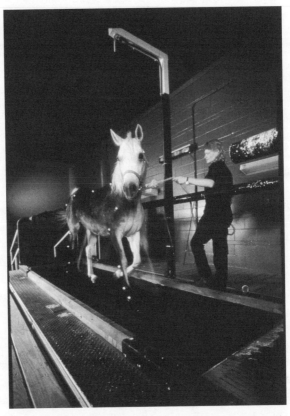

A lame horse is evaluated on a treadmill at the Equine Hospital at the University of Missouri's College of Veterinary Medicine.

North Carolina State University

Student Services Office
College of Veterinary Medicine
4700 Hillsborough Street, Box 8401
North Carolina State University
Raleigh NC 27606
Telephone: (919) 513-6262
Email: ncsucvmdvm@ncsu.edu
www.cvm.ncsu.edu

The North Carolina State College of Veterinary Medicine is located on a 182-acre site in Raleigh, the state capital, which has a population of more than 300,000. The sandy shores of North Carolina's beautiful coastline are a short ride to the east, and the Great Smoky Mountains are to the west. The climate includes mild winters and warm summers.

The College of Veterinary Medicine opened in the fall of 1981 and occupies more than 260,000 square feet, including a teaching hospital, classrooms, animal wards, research and teaching laboratories, and an audiovisual area. The college has 120 faculty members and a capacity for 304 veterinary medical students with training for interns, residents, and graduate students.

Construction started fall 2002 on the Centennial Biomedical Campus, which will be anchored by the College of Veterinary Medicine. An extension of the original NCSU Centennial Campus concept, the Centennial Biomedical Campus will house approximately 32 building sites. It will include an additional 1.6 million square feet of space over the next 25 years, resulting in a five-fold expansion of the current college and teaching hospital.

The Centennial Biomedical Campus will emphasize partnerships that work to bring academia, government and industry together. The focus of this campus is on biomedical applications, both to animals and humans. It will provide opportunities for industry and government researchers, entrepreneurs, clinical trial companies, as well as collaborations with other universities to work side by side with faculty and students at the College of Veterinary Medicine.

Application Information

For specific application information (availability, deadlines, fees, and VMCAS participation), please refer to the contact information listed above.

Residency implications: priority is given to North Carolina residents. There are approximately 14 nonresident positions.

Prerequisites for Admission

Course requirements and semester hours

English composition I, plus either English composition II, public speaking, or communication	6
College calculus	3
Introduction to statistics	3
General physics I, II (with laboratory)	8
General chemistry I, II (with laboratory)	8
Organic chemistry I, II (with laboratory)	8
General biology (with laboratory)	4
Principles of genetics	4
General microbiology (with laboratory)	4
Biochemistry	3
Social sciences and humanities	6
Business/finance	6

AP credit policy: must appear on official college transcripts and be equivalent to the appropriate college-level coursework.

Course completion deadline: only 2 courses may be pending completion in the spring semester, and both must be completed (with transcript evidence) by the end of the spring semester prior to matriculation. Pending courses (including correspondence courses) may not be completed in the summer session immediately preceding matriculation.

Standardized examinations: Graduate Record Examination (GRE®), general test, is required. The scores must be received by the October 3 application deadline.

Additional requirements and considerations

Animal/veterinary knowledge, experience, motivation, and maturity
Personal statement
Recommendations/evaluations (3 required; at least 2 from
     veterinarians/scientists with whom applicant has worked)
Extracurricular activities

Summary of Admission Procedure

Timetable

Application deadline: October 3
Date acceptances mailed: by April 1
School begins: August

Deposit (to hold place in class): $250.00.

Deferments: are considered for 1 year only, subject to Admissions Committee approval.

Evaluation criteria
Selection for admission is a 2-phase process:
Phase 1—Objective criteria:
    Required course GPA
    Cumulative GPA
    GPA in last 45+ credits attempted
    Test score
    Supplemental application

Phase 2—Subjective score:
    Applicant folder review by admissions committee

2004–2005 admissions summary

	Number of Applicants	Number of New Entrants*
Resident	194	62
Nonresident	370	14
Total:	564	76

* Estimated

Expenses for the 2004–2005 Academic Year

Tuition and fees (estimated)

Resident	$9,831.00
Nonresident	$32,594.00

Dual Degree Programs

Combined DVM–graduate degree programs are available.

Early Admission Program

Two special admissions options are available: (1) for North Carolina residents focusing on swine, poultry, or food animal medicine in concert with the College of Agriculture and Life Sciences, and (2) for students focusing on laboratory animal medicine in concert with the College of Agriculture at North Carolina A&T State University.

The Ohio State University

Chairperson, Admissions Committee
College of Veterinary Medicine
Suite 127 Veterinary Medicine Academic Building
1900 Coffey Road
The Ohio State University
Columbus OH 43210-1089
Telephone: (614) 292-8831
Fax: (614) 292-6989
Email: sander.28@osu.edu
www.vet.osu.edu

Ohio State University is located in Columbus, the capital of Ohio. Columbus is a congregation of cities and villages with a sense of history and a friendly atmosphere. The third-ranking center of scientific and technological research and data dissemination in the United States, the city offers fine arts, restaurants, sports, architecture, nature, community festivals, churches, and other areas of interest.

The Ohio State University is one of the nation's leading academic centers, with a sprawling campus straddling the Olentangy River. The campus consists of thousands of acres, hundreds of buildings, more than 15,000 faculty and staff, and more than 54,000 students. The veterinary college is the third-oldest in the United States and is one of the largest veterinary colleges in North America. The patient load is one of the highest in the country, and farmlands can be accessed 10 miles from campus. The faculty members have diverse academic and research activities, and 85 percent of the clinical teaching faculty are board certified. The academic curriculum is a 4-year program that blends some clinical experience into the first 2 years, while the last 2 years are mostly clinical.

Application Information

For specific application information (availability, deadlines, fees, and VMCAS participation), please refer to the contact information listed above.

Residency implications: priority is given to Ohio residents. Ohio contracts with West Virginia (5). Ohio will consider qualified nonresident students.

Prerequisites for Admission

For the humanities and social sciences requirement, students are encouraged to elect the courses required for the bachelor of science curriculum. Courses in communication, journalism, sociology, economics, and animal behavior are strongly recommended.

Students enrolled in the preveterinary medicine curriculum are encouraged to take electives that will provide a well-rounded education in addition to those biological sciences preparatory to the veterinary medical curriculum.

Course requirements and quarter hours

English	5
General chemistry (with laboratory)*	15
Organic chemistry*	6
Biochemistry*	5
Biology*	10
Genetics*	5
Microbiology (with laboratory)*	5
Mathematics (algebra and trigonometry)	5
General physics (with laboratory)*	10
Humanities and social sciences	20
Electives	10

* Must have been completed within the 10 years preceding the application deadline.

Graduate students must have a letter from their advisor releasing them from their graduate program if accepted into the veterinary medicine program.

Required undergraduate GPA: the minimum acceptable GPA for Ohio residents is 2.80; however, students with 3.00 average or above will be given preferential consideration. The minimum acceptable GPA for contract-state residents is 3.00 and for nonresidents is 3.40 (on a 4.00 scale). An undergraduate degree is not a requirement. A single, comprehensive GPA, which will include grades from all college-level work (both graduate and undergraduate) completed by the applicant, is calculated.

AP credit policy: AP credit given.

Course completion deadline: all but one prerequisite course must be completed by the end of the fall semester or quarter coinciding with submission of the application. The final remaining prerequisite course must be completed at the end of the following term (spring semester or winter quarter). Failure to satisfactorily complete all prerequisites with a grade of C or better will result in automatic loss of a candidate's seat in the class.

Standardized examinations: Scores from one of the following standardized examinations must be submitted at the time of application:

> *Graduate Record Examination (GRE®)*: minimum acceptable score 955 total of all three subtests.
>
> *Medical College Admission Test (MCAT)*: minimum acceptable score 24 total; score O-T on essay portion (new MCAT).
>
> *Veterinary College Admission Test (VCAT)*: minimum acceptable score 50th percentile.

Scores must not be older than five years prior to the application year. The most recent acceptable date for taking the examination is September 30 of the application year.

Additional requirements and considerations

> Minimum of 80 hours work with a veterinarian (volunteer or paid)
> Academic improvement/difficulty
> Personal evaluations
> Involvement in community affairs
> Communication/interpersonal skills
> Initiative/leadership
> Attitude/motivation/judgment
> Work record/financial responsibility
> Social and personal support systems
> Comprehensiveness of veterinary medical/animal work experience
> Comparative medical experience

Summary of Admission Procedure

Timetable

> Application deadline: October 2
> Date interviews are held: November–March
> Date acceptances mailed: December–March
> School begins: late September

Deposit (to hold place in class): $25.00 for residents; $300.00 for contract and nonresident applicants.

Deferments: not considered.

Evaluation criteria

	% weight
Grades	35
Test scores	10
Interview*	55

* Preferred applicants are interviewed and evaluated by members of the Admissions Committee. The academic interview covers subjective areas such as academic improvement

versus difficulty, communication/interpersonal skills, involvement in social and community activities, social and personal support systems, work record/financial responsibility, motivation and commitment to veterinary medicine, comprehension of veterinary medicine, knowledge of and/or exposure to animals, and references. Those applicants given the highest overall evaluation are selected for the entering class.

2005–2006 admissions summary

	Number of Applicants	Number of New Entrants
Resident	273	100
Contract*	15	5
Nonresident	585	35
Total:	873	140

Expenses for the 2005–2006 Academic Year

Tuition and fees

Resident	$17,955.00
Nonresident*†	$44,691.00

* For further information, see the listing of contracting states and provinces.

† Contract students are assessed the nonresident tuition and fees. The contract state subsidy is subtracted from that tuition, and the student pays the balance due.

Dual-Degree Programs

Combined DVM–graduate degree programs are available.

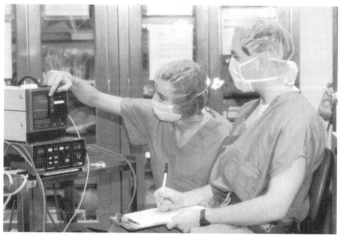

Veterinary students monitor the vital signs of a patient during surgery at the North Carolina State University Veterinary Teaching Hospital. Photo courtesy of North Carolina State University College of Veterinary Medicine.

Oklahoma State University

Office of Admissions
112 McElroy Hall
Center for Veterinary Health Sciences
College of Veterinary Medicine
Oklahoma State University
Stillwater OK 74078-2003
Telephone: (405) 744-6961 or (405) 744-6653
Fax: (405) 744-0356
Email: robin.wilson@okstate.edu
www.cvhs.okstate.edu

Oklahoma State University is located in Stillwater, which has a population of about 39,000. Stillwater is in north central Oklahoma about 65 miles from Oklahoma City and 69 miles from Tulsa. The campus is exceptionally beautiful, with modified Georgian-style architecture in the new buildings. It encompasses 840 acres and more than 60 major academic buildings.

Three major buildings form the veterinary medicine complex. The oldest, McElroy Hall, houses the William E. Brock Memorial Library and Learning Center, as well as new classrooms and laboratories. The Boren Veterinary Medical Teaching Hospital provides modern facilities for both academic and clinical instruction. Completing the triad is the Oklahoma Animal Disease Diagnostic Laboratory, which provides teaching resources for students in the professional curriculum and diagnostic services to Oklahoma agriculture and industry. The College of Veterinary Medicine is fully accredited by the American Veterinary Medical Association. Faculty members in the 3 academic departments share responsibility for the curriculum. These departments are Veterinary Clinical Sciences, Veterinary Pathobiology, and Physiological Sciences.

Application Information

For specific application information (availability, deadlines, fees, and VMCAS participation), please refer to the contact information listed above.

Residency implications: priority is given to Oklahoma residents. Nonresidents may apply, and Oklahoma State could admit up to 4 contract students from New Jersey and up to 20 first-time nonresident students (including any contract students from Arkansas or Delaware).

Prerequisites for Admission

Course requirements and semester hours

English composition	6
English elective	3
General chemistry (with laboratory)	8–10
Organic chemistry (with laboratory)	5–8
Biochemistry	3
Physics	8
Mathematics	3
Zoology (with laboratory)	4
Animal nutrition	3
Biological science elective	3
Microbiology (with laboratory)	4–5
Genetics (laboratory recommended)	3–4
Humanities or social sciences	6
Electives (science or business)	2

Required undergraduate GPA: a minimum GPA of 2.80 on a 4.00 scale is required in prerequisite courses. The mean cumulative GPA of the 2005 entering class was 3.509.

AP credit policy: AP credit accepted if documented on college transcript.

Alternative admissions: the Oklahoma State Regents for Higher Education permit the college to accept up to 15 percent of a beginning class who do not meet minimum requirements (contact admissions office for criteria).

Course completion deadline: prerequisite courses must be completed by the end of the spring semester just prior to matriculation.

Standardized examinations: Graduate Record Examination (GRE®), general test and biology subject test, is required. Earliest acceptable test date is June 2002. The class of 2009 had mean scores of 488 verbal, 635 quantitative, and 590 biology.

Additional requirements and considerations
   Evidence of motivation over an extended period of time
   Animal/veterinary work experience
   Amount of undergraduate education completed
   Recommendations/evaluations (3 required)
      Veterinarian (required)
      Academic advisor, preferred
      Employer
   Demonstrated leadership and interpersonal skills

All science courses must have been taken within 8 years of application (fall 1998 for class applying fall 2006)

Summary of Admission Procedure

Timetable

Application deadline: October 2
Date interviews held: February
Date acceptances mailed: March
School begins: mid- to late August

Deposit (to hold place in class): resident, $100.00; nonresident, $500.00.

Deferments: to complete graduate degree, deferments are considered.

Evaluation criteria

The admission procedure consists of evaluation of both academic and non-academic criteria. The Admissions Committee considers all factors in the applicant's file, but the following are especially important: academic achievement; familiarity with the profession and sincerity of interest; recommendations; test scores; extracurricular activities; character, personality, and general fitness and commitment for a career in veterinary medicine. The committee selects those applicants considered most capable of excelling as veterinary medical students and who possess the greatest potential for success in the veterinary medical profession.

2005–2006 admissions summary

	Number of Applicants	Number of New Entrants
Resident	129	56
Nonresident	270	24
Total:	399	80

Expenses for the 2004–2005 Academic Year

Tuition and fees

Resident	$11,500.00
Nonresident	$29,000.00

Dual-Degree Programs

Combined DVM–graduate degree programs are available.

Oregon State University

Office of the Dean
College of Veterinary Medicine
Oregon State University
200 Magruder Hall
Corvallis OR 97331-4801
Telephone: (541) 737-2098
Fax: (541) 737-4245
Email: cvmproginfo@oregonstate.edu
www.vet.oregonstate.edu

At Oregon State University's College of Veterinary Medicine, students learn the skills to treat and prevent animal diseases through a rigorous course of study taught by a dedicated faculty.

The city of Corvallis, home of OSU, is a modern city of approximately 50,000 that boasts theaters and parks, an art center and shopping malls, and public transportation and bicycle paths to every corner of the community. Life in Corvallis includes lectures, concerts, films, and exhibits through the university. Students can explore the great outdoors just over an hour away by car at the spectacular Oregon coast, the snow-capped Oregon Cascades, and the city of Portland. In the heart of the agriculturally rich Willamette River Valley, Corvallis enjoys colorful and crisp autumns, mild and rainy winters, flowering springs, and warm, dry summers.

The new four-year DVM program began in the fall of 2003, with the entering class spending all four years at Oregon State University, in Corvallis, Oregon. The small class size of 48 helps to provide the students with an excellent veterinary education and the opportunity to have close interaction with faculty.

Application Information

For specific application information (availability, deadlines, fees, and VMCAS participation), please refer to the contact information listed above.

Residency implications: Oregon residents and WICHE-sponsored students are eligible for resident fees. A limited number of students are accepted as non-residents. Priority is given to Oregon students with 8 positions available to WICHE and all other non-resident applicants.

Prerequisites for Admission

Course requirements and quarter hours

Chemistry	A series of chemistry courses through upper-division biochemistry. This includes a sequence of inorganic chemistry courses with laboratories and organic chemistry sufficient to meet requirements for an upper-division biochemistry course or course sequence.
Biochemistry	A course or complete course sequence in upper-division biochemistry.
Mathematics	Sufficient to meet the prerequisite for physics and inorganic chemistry (at least college-level algebra)
Physics	2 quarters or 1 semester of college-level physics for science majors
Zoology or biology	1 year sequence
Genetics	1 quarter or semester of an upper-division course
Animal nutrition	1 quarter or 1 semester of a general animal nutrition course
Biological sciences	A minimum of at least 6 additional quarter hours or 4 semester hours of upper-division biological science courses, with at least one laboratory (physiology, cell physiology, cell biology, microbiology, or additional biochemistry)

Total minimum number of credits required: 120 quarter credits; 80 semester credits.

Required undergraduate GPA: overall GPA must be at least 3.00 or the last 2 years must be at least 3.00. Prerequisite courses taken after August 2004, other than AP credit, must be graded A–F. A student who attends an institution that traditionally does not provide grades will be evaluated on a case-by-case basis. The mean overall GPA for the class entering in fall of 2004 was 3.53.

AP credit policy: must appear on official college transcripts and be equivalent to the appropriate college-level coursework.

Course completion deadline: prerequisite courses must be completed by July 1 prior to entry.

Standardized examinations: Graduate Record Examination (GRE®), general test, is required. The test deadline for applicants to the entering class of 2007 is October 2, 2006. The mean score of the 2005 entering class was at the 54.66 percentile.

Additional requirements and considerations:

Those seeking admission to the College of Veterinary Medicine are expected to have a good understanding of the depth and breadth of the profession. Applicants should observe or work with veterinarians and confirm that they enjoy working with animals and are concerned for their health and welfare. Veterinary experience may be gained by working or volunteering in a research laboratory, clinical practice, animal shelter, zoo, animal rehabilitation facility, or public health, regulatory, or industrial setting.

Recommendations (3 required, one by a veterinarian)

Extracurricular and/or community service activities desirable

Summary of Admission Procedure

Timetable

Application deadline: October 2
Date interviews are held: late February
Date acceptances mailed: mid-March
School begins: late September

Deposit (to hold place in class): $50.00.

Deferments: are rare.

Evaluation criteria

The admission procedure consists of 2 parts: a file review and a personal interview of applicants considered to be competitive. (Interviews for nonresidents and WICHE students may not be required.)

	% weight
Grades	30
Test scores	6
Animal/veterinary experience	17
Interview	22
References, personal development	21
Academic index: quality and quantity of course load, work commitments, etc.	4

(Additional points may be awarded in a "diversity/adversity" category.)

2005–2006 admissions summary

	Number of Applicants	Number of New Entrants
Resident	96	40
Contract (WICHE)*	161	0
Nonresident	406	8
Total:	663	48

Expenses for the 2005–2006 Academic Year

Tuition and fees

Resident (approximate)	$14,850.00
Nonresident	
Contract*	$14,850.00
Other nonresident (approximate)	$28,323.00

* For further information, see the listing of contracting states and provinces.

Dual-Degree Programs

Combined DVM–graduate degree programs are available.

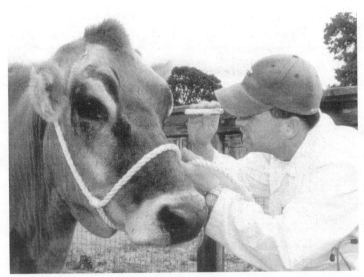

Up close and personal: with practice, students develop examination skills to deal with all sorts of patients. Photo courtesy of Oregon State University College of Veterinary Medicine.

University of Pennsylvania

Admissions Office
School of Veterinary Medicine
3800 Spruce Street
University of Pennsylvania
Philadelphia PA 19104-6044
Telephone: (215) 898-5434
Fax: (215) 573-8819
Email: admissions@vet.upenn.edu
www.vet.upenn.edu

The University of Pennsylvania is located in West Philadelphia. Philadelphia is a city with a strong cultural heritage. Independence National Park includes 1 square mile of historic Philadelphia next to the Delaware River. Included are Independence Hall, the Liberty Bell, and many fine examples of colonial architecture. Philadelphia also offers theaters, museums, sports, and outdoor recreation. The Philadelphia Zoo, first in the nation, houses more than 1,600 mammals, birds, reptiles, and amphibians. The School of Veterinary Medicine enjoys a close relationship with the zoo.

The School of Veterinary Medicine was founded in 1884 and includes a hospital for small animals, classrooms, and research facilities in the city. The large-animal hospital and research facilities are located at the New Bolton Center, an 800-acre farm 40 miles west of Philadelphia. The first 2 years are spent on the main campus. Part of the third year may be spent at the New Bolton Center, and the fourth year is spent in rotation and on electives at varying campus locations. Off-campus electives are frequently permitted.

Application Information

For specific application information (availability, deadlines, fees, and VMCAS participation), please refer to the contact information listed above.

Residency implications: priority is given to Pennsylvania residents. Contract arrangements are with New Jersey. The number of nonresident places is usually 40–45, including international applicants.

Prerequisites for Admission

At least 3 English credits must be in composition; biology courses must provide background in genetics. Organic chemistry must cover aliphatic and aromatic compounds to fulfill the requirement.

Course requirements and semester hours

English (including composition)	6
Physics (with laboratory)	8
Chemistry (with at least 1 laboratory)	
General	8
Organic	4
Biology or zoology (3 courses)	9
Social sciences or humanities	6
Calculus	3
Electives	46

(Although not required, biochemistry is strongly recommended.)

Required undergraduate GPA: no specific GPA. Applicants are evaluated comparatively and should have at least a GPA of 3.30 to be competitive. The mean cumulative GPA of the class admitted in 2004 was 3.50.

AP credit policy: must appear on official college transcripts and count toward degree.

Course completion deadline: prerequisite courses must be completed by the end of the summer term of the year in which admission is sought.

Standardized examinations: Graduate Record Examination (GRE®), general test, is required; the GRE Code for Pennvet is 2775. Test scores should be received no later than November 1. The class admitted in 2004 had an average of 580 on the verbal subtest and 720 on the quantitative subtest.

Additional requirements and considerations
 Animal/veterinary work experience: experience working with animals, direct veterinary work, or research experience is desired. No minimum time limit. Experience should be sufficient to convince the admissions committee of motivation, interest, and understanding.
 Recommendations/evaluations: 3 required, one from an academic science source; and one from a veterinarian. The third is the choice of the applicant.
 Extracurricular/community service activities: additional activities in this category can provide information important to the admissions committee.
 Leadership: evidence of leadership abilities is desirable.

Summary of Admission Procedure

Timetable

> Application deadline: October 2
> Date interviews are held: Fridays from late January until completion
> Date acceptances mailed: within 14 days after interview
> School begins: early September

Deposit (to hold place in class): $500.00.

Deferments: are considered on an individual basis.

Evaluation criteria

The seats are filled through a 2-part admission procedure, which includes a file review and personal interviews.

> Grades
> Test scores
> Animal/veterinary experience
> Interview
> References
> Essay
> English skills (TOEFL)

File review: files are reviewed in January by pairs of members of the admissions committee (including an alumni member), and decisions are made on whether or not to offer an interview.

Personal interviews: interviews are held on Fridays from late January until the class is filled. The number of interviews granted equals 1½ to 2 times the number of seats available.

Two personal interviews are conducted: a formal interview with 2 faculty members (including an alumni member) of the committee, and an informal interview with student committee members. Although students do not vote on acceptance, they have a significant part in the meeting following interviews.

2005–2006 admissions summary

	Number of Applicants	Number of New Entrants
Resident	229	63
Nonresident*	1,022	45
Total:	1,251	108

* For further information, see listing of contracting states and provinces.

Expenses for the 2005–2006 Academic Year

Tuition and fees

Resident	$28,998.00
Nonresident	
Contract*	$28,998.00
Other nonresident	$34,470.00

* For further information, see listing of contracting states and provinces.

Dual-Degree Programs

Combined VMD–graduate degree programs are available.

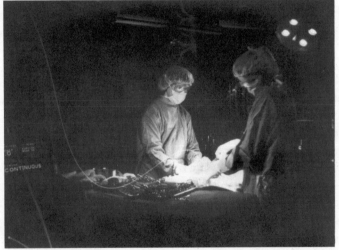

Veterinarians at Oklahoma State University's College of Veterinary Medicine perform laser surgery as part of their investigation of the medical application of lasers. Photo courtesy of the College of Veterinary Medicine, Oklahoma State University.

Purdue University

Student Services Office
School of Veterinary Medicine
625 Harrison Street
Purdue University
West Lafayette IN 47907-2026
Telephone: (765) 494-7893 or (800) 213-2859 (long distance)
Email: vetadmissions@purdue.edu
www.vet.purdue.edu/admissions

Purdue University is located in one of the largest metropolitan centers in northwestern Indiana. Greater Lafayette occupies a site on the Wabash River 65 miles northwest of Indianapolis and 126 miles southeast of Chicago. The combined population of the twin cities, Lafayette and West Lafayette, exceeds 64,000. The community offers an art museum, historical museum, 1,600 acres of public parks, and more than 60 churches of all major denominations.

Purdue ranks among the 25 largest colleges and universities in the nation. Students represent all 50 states and many foreign countries. Diversity and opportunity are goals that the School of Veterinary Medicine maintains in the selection of each year's entering class. The School of Veterinary Medicine has assumed a leading position nationally and internationally in veterinary education. To better prepare individuals for veterinary medical careers in the twenty-first century, new and innovative strategies have been incorporated into the curriculum.

Application Information

For specific application information (availability, deadlines, fees, and VMCAS participation), please refer to the contact information listed above.

Residency implications: priority is given to Indiana residents. Approximately one-third of the class will be nonresident students in a total class of 60. Applicants from all states will be considered. Purdue has no contract positions. International applicants will be considered provided both the academic and financial criteria can be met.

Prerequisites for Admission

The course requirements outlined below are considered the bare minimum prerequisite courses to be completed. No less than a grade of C must be received in each required course in order to be considered eligible for admission. In the electives category, humanities include languages, cognitive sciences, and social sciences. Other courses are highly recommended and can be found on our website.

Course requirements and number of semesters

Inorganic chemistry with lab	2
Organic chemistry with lab	2
Biochemistry	1
Biology with lab (diversity, developmental, cell structure)	2
Genetics with lab	1
Microbiology (general or medical) with lab	1
Nutrition (animal)	1
Physics with lab	2
Calculus	1
Statistics	1
English composition	1
Communication (interpersonal, persuasion or speech)	1
Careers in Veterinary Medicine (if available)	1
Humanities (foreign languages, cognitive sciences, and social sciences)	3

Note: Complete course sequences should be followed rather than focusing on credit hours.

Required undergraduate GPA: the mean cumulative GPA of the 2005 entering class was 3.60 on a 4.00 scale. The minimum overall GPA required for consideration is 3.00 on a 4.00 scale for nonresident applicants.

AP credit policy: must appear on official college transcripts by subject area and be equivalent to the appropriate college-level coursework.

Course completion deadline: minimum prerequisite courses must be completed by the end of the spring term prior to matriculation.

Standardized examinations: Graduate Record Examination (GRE®), general test, is required. Test scores must be received no later than November 1 of the year of application.

Additional requirements and considerations

Animal/veterinary experience
Amount of college education
Recommendations/evaluations (3 required)
    Academic advisor/faculty member
    Employer
    Veterinarian

Essay
Employment record
Extracurricular college experience

Summary of Admission Procedure

Timetable

Application deadline: October 2
Date interviews are held: February
Date acceptances mailed: March
School begins: late August

Deposit (to hold place in class): $250.00 for residents; $1,000.00 for nonresidents.

Deferments: request for deferments will be considered on a case-by-case basis.

Evaluation criteria

The admission process consists of:

A preliminary review based upon grade point indices, test scores, and prerequisite course completion
An in-depth review of selected applicants
A personal interview by invitation

	% weight
Grades, test scores, overall academic performance	54
Animal, veterinary, and general work experiences, extracurricular activities, essay, overall presentation of application materials, references, and interview	46

2005–2006 admissions summary

	Number of Applicants	Number of New Entrants
Resident	104	43
Nonresident	463	23
International	7	2
Total:	574	68

Expenses for the 2005–2006 Academic Year

Tuition and fees

Resident	$13,352.00
Nonresident	$32,188.00

Dual-Degree Programs

Combined DVM–graduate degree programs are available.

Early Admission Program

The Veterinary Scholars Program provides an opportunity for early admission into the professional program by accepting high-school seniors who

1. ranked in the top 10 percent of their graduating class;
2. have attained a combined SAT score equal to or greater than 1950 or composite ACT score equal to or greater than 28;
3. were admitted to Purdue University and committed to a major in animal sciences, biochemistry, or biological sciences programs; and
4. demonstrate a background of work experience with animals and veterinarians.

Students admitted to the program must complete all preveterinary prerequisite coursework, obtain a bachelor's degree with stipulated grade point averages for each year of undergraduate study, and submit scores from the GRE® (Graduate Record Exam), general test, during their senior year.

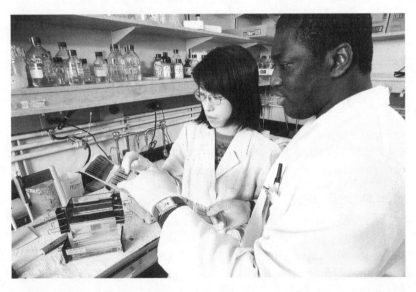

Many veterinary medical students choose a career in research rather than a clinical practice. Photo by Vincent P. Walter, courtesy of Purdue University.

University of Tennessee

Admissions Office
College of Veterinary Medicine
2407 River Drive
Room A-104-C
Knoxville TN 37996-4550
Telephone: (865) 974-7354
Email: dshepherd@utk.edu
www.vet.utk.edu

The University of Tennessee's College of Veterinary Medicine is located in Knoxville, a city of 185,000 situated in the Appalachian foothills of east central Tennessee. Only 45 minutes from the Great Smoky Mountains National Park and 3 hours from both Nashville and Atlanta, Knoxville offers many recreational and cultural opportunities, including a symphony orchestra, an opera company, and several fine theaters. The climate in Knoxville is moderate with distinct seasons.

The 417-acre Knoxville campus of the University of Tennessee has about 19,500 undergraduate and 6,000 graduate students. The modern Clyde M. York Veterinary Medicine Building, housing the teaching and research facilities, Veterinary Teaching Hospital, and Agriculture-Veterinary Medicine Library, faces the Tennessee River on the university's Agricultural Campus.

The curriculum of the College of Veterinary Medicine is a 9-semester, 4-year program. Development of a strong basic science education is emphasized in the first year. The second and third years emphasize the study of diseases, their causes, diagnosis, treatment, and prevention. Innovative features of this curriculum include 6 weeks of student-centered small-group applied-learning exercises in semesters 1–5; 3 weeks of dedicated clinical experiences in the veterinary teaching hospital in semesters 3–5; and elective course opportunities in semesters 4–9 that allow students to focus on specific educational/career goals. In the fourth year (final 3 semesters), students participate exclusively in clinical rotations in the Veterinary Teaching Hospital and in required off-campus externships. The college has unique programs in zoo and exotic animal medicine and surgery, cancer diagnosis and therapy, endoscopy, laser surgery, and rehabilitation/physical therapy.

Application Information

For specific application information (availability, deadlines, fees, and VMCAS participation), please refer to the contact information listed above.

Residency implications: priority is given to Tennessee residents. Tennessee has no contractual agreements and does accept nonresident applications.

Prerequisites for Admission

Course requirements and semester hours

General inorganic chemistry (with laboratory)	8
Organic chemistry (with laboratory)	8
General biology/zoology (with laboratory)	8
Cellular biology*	3
Genetics	3
Biochemistry (exclusive of laboratory)[†]	4
Physics (with laboratory)	8
English composition	6
Social sciences/humanities	18

* Applicants are strongly encouraged to complete additional biological and physical science courses, especially comparative anatomy, mammalian physiology, microbiology with laboratory, and statistics.

† This should be a complete upper-division course in general cellular and comparative biochemistry. Half of a 2-semester sequence will not satisfy this requirement.

AP credit policy: must appear on official college transcripts and be equivalent to the appropriate college-level coursework.

Required undergraduate GPA: for nonresident applicants, the minimum acceptable cumulative GPA is 3.20 on a 4.00 scale. At time of acceptance, the mean GPA of the class entering in fall of 2005 was 3.59.

Course completion deadline: prerequisite courses must be completed with a grade of C or better by the end of the spring term prior to entry.

Standardized examinations: Graduate Record Exam (GRE®), general test, is required. For applicants planning to matriculate in August 2007, the oldest acceptable GRE scores are from the November 1, 2002, test date.

Additional requirements and considerations

Animal/veterinary work experience
Recommendations/evaluations
Extracurricular and/or community service activities
Leadership skills
Autobiographical essay (personal statement)

Summary of Admission Procedure

Timetable

    Application deadline: October 2
    Date interviews are held: mid- to late March
    Date acceptances mailed: no later than April 1
    Applicant's response date: April 15
    School begins: late August

Deposit (to hold place in class): none required.

Deferments: are considered on a case-by-case basis.

Evaluation criteria

The admission procedure consists of an initial file review followed by an interview of selected applicants.

    Initial academic file review:
      Grades
      Test scores
    Animal/veterinary experience
    Interview
    References (3 required)
    Essay

2004–2005 admissions summary

	Number of Applicants	Number of New Entrants
Resident	128	51
Nonresident	637	19
Total:	765	70

Expenses for the 2005–2006 Academic Year

Tuition and fees

Resident	$11,612.00
Nonresident	$32,578.00

Parallel Degree Program

The College, in partnership with the College of Education, Health and Human Sciences, offers an option for veterinary students (and graduate veterinarians) to earn the MPH degree with a concentration in Veterinary Public Health. Contact the College of Veterinary Medicine for additional information.

Texas A & M University

Office of the Dean
Attn: Student Admissions
College of Veterinary Medicine
Texas A & M University
College Station TX 77843-4461
Telephone: (979) 862-1169
www.cvm.tamu.edu

The university is located adjacent to the cities of Bryan and College Station. The two cities have a combined population of about 100,000. The student population at Texas A & M is more than 40,000. The College of Veterinary Medicine is one of the 10 original veterinary teaching institutions that existed in the United States prior to World War II.

The College provides an integrated professional curriculum that prepares graduates with a firm foundation in the basic sciences, a broad comparative medicine knowledge base, and the clinical and personal skills to be leaders in the many career fields of veterinary medicine. Professional students are given the opportunity to gain additional education and training in their personal career paths.

Becoming a veterinarian requires much dedication and diligent study. The veterinary medical student is required to meet a high level of performance. The demands on students' time and effort are considerable, but the rewards and career satisfaction are personal achievements that make significant contributions to our society.

Application Information

For specific application information (availability, deadlines, fees, and VMCAS participation), please refer to the contact information listed above.

Residency implications: Texas has no contractual agreements with other states. Applicants from other states who have outstanding credentials will be considered. Successful candidates who are awarded competitive university-based scholarships may attend at resident tuition rate.

Prerequisites for Admission

The minimum number of college or university credits required for admission into the professional curriculum is 70 semester hours. Applicants must have completed or have in progress approximately 54 credit hours at the time of application. Because there is no specific degree plan associated with preveterinary education, students are encouraged to pursue a degree plan that meets individual interests. Students are strongly encouraged to choose courses with the assistance of a knowledgeable counselor at the undergraduate institution or through contact with an academic advisor at the College of Veterinary Medicine, telephone: (979) 862-1169.

Course requirements and semester hours (subject to change)

Life sciences

General biology (with laboratory)   4
Survey of contemporary biology that covers the chemical basis of life, structure and biology of the cell, molecular biology, and genetics

General microbiology (with laboratory)   4
Basic microbiology; comparative morphology, taxonomy, pathogenesis, ecology, variation, and physiology of microorganisms

Genetics   3
Basic concepts of mammalian genetics

Animal nutrition or feeds and feeding   3
Emphasis on basic principles of animal nutrition; nutritional roles of carbohydrates, proteins, lipids, minerals, vitamins, and water; emphasis on digestion, absorption, metabolism, and excretion of the nutrients and their metabolites

Chemical-physical sciences and mathematics

Inorganic chemistry (with laboratory)   8
Basic concepts of modern inorganic chemistry

Organic chemistry (with laboratory)   8
Basic concepts of modern organic chemistry

Biochemistry   5
An introduction to the chemistry and metabolism of biologically important molecules, the biochemical basis of life processes, and cellular metabolism and regulation

Calculus/statistics   3

Physics (with laboratory)   8
Fundamentals of mechanics, heat, sound, electricity, and light

Nonscience

Composition and rhetoric   3
Literature   3
Speech communication   3
Technical writing   3

Additional credits

In addition to the 58 credit hours recommended above, an applicant must complete a minimum of 12 additional credits. Applicants should keep in mind their degree program, the core curriculum requirements for a baccalaureate degree at Texas A & M University, and their personal career goals in making these choices. Applicants are strongly encouraged to make these choices with a qualified counselor at their institution.

Required undergraduate GPA: the minimum overall GPA required is 2.90 on a 4.00 scale or 3.10 for the last 45 semester credits. The mean of the most recent entering class was 3.64.

AP credit policy: AP credit is accepted as fulfilling selected prerequisites; credit must be reflected on the official undergraduate transcript.

Course completion deadline: required courses must be completed by the end of the spring term prior to entry.

Standardized examinations: Graduate Record Examination (GRE®), general test, is required. Beginning October 3, 2002, all applicants applying for fall 2004 entry and beyond are required to take the general test of the GRE (which includes the analytical writing section).

Additional requirements and considerations

Evaluations

Animal/veterinary work experience

Knowledge and experience in working with animals is crucial to becoming a successful veterinarian. While the professional curriculum is almost totally devoted to the understanding of animals, animal contact, experience, and handling should also be major considerations in the preveterinary training period. Applicants are expected to be familiar with animal systems and behavior. For those interested in food supply veterinary medicine, general agriculture knowledge should also be a consideration. To obtain this experience, applicants should either register for coursework based on their background, interests, and needs, or involve themselves in practical animal operations. Formal training in animal systems and animal behavior is highly desirable and encouraged if available at the applicant's institution.

Summary of Admission Procedure

Timetable

Application deadline: October 1
Date interviews are held: December–mid-February
Date acceptances mailed: mid-March
School begins: late August

Deposit (to hold place in class): none required.

Deferments: requests for deferments will be considered on a case-by-case basis.

Evaluation criteria

Academic performance
Test scores
Interview
Personal statement
Personal evaluations (3 evaluations are required)
Semester course load and postacademic challenge
Leadership and experience

2005–2006 admissions summary

	Number of Applicants	Number of New Entrants
Resident	302	123
Nonresident	102	9
Total:	404	132

Expenses for the 2005–2006 Academic Year

Tuition and fees

Resident	$11,410.00
Nonresident	$22,750.00

Tufts University

Office of Admissions
Cummings School of Veterinary Medicine
200 Westboro Road
Tufts University
North Grafton MA 01536
Telephone: (508) 839-7920
Email: vetadmissions@tufts.edu
www.tufts.edu/vet/

Tufts University is located near Boston, where athletic and cultural activities abound. The Cummings School of Veterinary Medicine provides an exciting biomedical environment for the study of modern veterinary medicine. Signature programs include wildlife medicine, equine sports medicine, international veterinary medicine, biotechnology and veterinary medicine, and the study of issues related to ethical dimensions of veterinary medicine, including animal welfare. Hands-on learning begins in the first year and continues throughout the next 3 years. Many opportunities exist outside of formal courses for hands-on work in hospitals and research laboratories. The Hospital for Large Animals, Foster Hospital for Small Animals, the Ambulatory Clinic, and the Bernice Barbour Wildlife Clinic provide a rich mixture of horses, cats, dogs, cattle, sheep, goats, and native wildlife.

Application Information

For specific application information (availability, deadlines, fees, and VMCAS participation), please refer to the contact information listed above.

Residency implications: Massachusetts residents make up about half of each class. All others considered for the remaining spaces. Tufts contracts with Maine (1), New Hampshire (1–2), and New Jersey (4).

Prerequisites for Admission

Course requirements and semesters

Biology (with laboratory)	2
Inorganic chemistry (with laboratory)	2
Organic chemistry (with laboratory)	2
Physics	2
Mathematics	2
Genetics, unless included in biology	1
Biochemistry	1
English composition	2
Social and behavioral sciences	2
Humanities and fine arts	2

Required undergraduate GPA: no minimum GPA required. The average GPA for the class admitted in 2005 was 3.63.

AP credit policy: must appear on official college transcripts and be equivalent to the appropriate college-level coursework.

Course completion deadline: prerequisite courses must be completed by the time of matriculation into the DVM program.

Standardized examinations: Graduate Record Examination (GRE®), general test, is required. The most recent acceptable test date for applicants to the class of 2011 is November 2006. The oldest acceptable scores must be within 5 years of the application deadline. Average GRE scores for the class of 2009 were verbal 600, quantitative 710, and analytical 5.0.

Additional requirements and considerations

Animal/veterinary/biomedical research experience
Evaluations (3 required)
    advisor/faculty members
    veterinarian/research scientist
Essays
Interview

Summary of Admission Procedure

Timetable

Application deadline: November 1
Date interviews are held: February
Date acceptances mailed: March
School begins: late August

Deposit (to hold place in class): $500.00.

Deferments: requests for deferment are handled on a case-by-case basis.

Evaluation criteria
Tufts' admission procedure consists of a review of the application and an interview of selected applicants.

2005–2006 admissions summary

	Number of Applicants	Number of New Entrants
Total:	715	80

Expenses for the 2004–2005 Academic Year

Tuition and fees

Resident	$28,855.00
Contract*	$21,947.00
Nonresident	$33,947.00

* For further information, see the listing of contracting states and provinces.

Dual-Degree Program

Combined DVM–graduate degree programs are available.

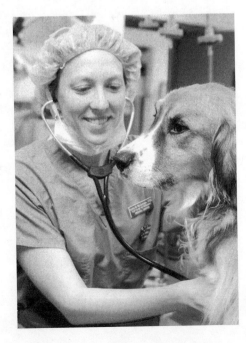

Veterinary medical students find their clinical rounds not only educational but also personally satisfying. Photo courtesy of Tufts University Cummings School of Veterinary Medicine.

Tuskegee University

Office of Veterinary Admissions
School of Veterinary Medicine, Nursing, and Allied Health
Tuskegee University
Tuskegee AL 36088
Telephone: (334) 727-8460

Tuskegee University School of Veterinary Medicine is located in Tuskegee, Alabama, a city of about 25,000. Tuskegee is located about 40 miles east of Montgomery and 40 miles west of Columbus, Georgia. Summers are hot and humid, and winters are moderate. Numerous lakes, parks, recreational facilities, and other educational institutions are located nearby.

The university was founded by Booker T. Washington in 1881, and the veterinary school was established in 1945. Over 70% of African-American veterinarians in the United States received their professional training at Tuskegee. A large portion of the campus has been declared a historical site by the National Park Service.

Application Information

For specific application information (availability, deadlines, fees, and VMCAS participation), please refer to the contact information listed above.

Residency implications: applications are accepted with special consideration given to Alabama residents. A minimum number of contract spaces are available for Kentucky (2), New Jersey (2), South Carolina (4), and West Virginia (2).

Prerequisites for Admission

Course requirements and semester hours

English composition/communications	6
Mathematics (algebra and trigonometry)	6
Chemistry (minimum)	
Organic chemistry (with laboratory)	4
Biochemistry (with laboratory)	4
Physics* (with laboratories)	8
Biological science	
Advanced biology**	9
Free electives	8
(advanced biological science—optional)	
Animal science	9
(includes poultry and animal nutrition)	
Social science and humanities	6
Electives—liberal arts	6

* One academic year

** Advanced biology courses, e.g., zoology, microbiology, genetics, anatomy, physiology, and histology

Required undergraduate GPA: the cumulative and science GPA requirement is 2.70 on a 4.00 scale.

AP credit policy: acceptable for English composition and mathematics.

Course completion deadline: prerequisite courses must be completed by the end of the spring semester of the year of application.

Standardized examinations: Medical College Admission Test (MCAT) or Graduate Record Examination (GRE®), any of which must be taken within 3 years of application, is required.

Summary of Admission Procedure

Timetable

    Application deadline: First Monday in December
    Date interviews are held: February–March
    Date acceptances mailed: April 15
    School begins: late August

Deposit (to hold place in class): $301.50.

Deferments: one-year deferments are considered on a case-by-case basis.

Evaluation criteria

The following items are taken into consideration: academic record, academic trends, letters of recommendation, work experience, and test scores.

	% weight
Grades	60
Test scores	2
Animal/veterinary experience	1
Interview	15
References	1
Essay	1

2002–2003 admissions summary

	Number of Applicants	*Number of New Entrants*
Resident	39	4
Contract*	80	15
Nonresident	139	41
Total:	258	60

Expenses for the 2002–2003 Academic Year

Tuition and fees

$12,000.00

* For further information, see the listing of contracting states and provinces.

Dual-Degree Programs

Combined DVM–graduate degree programs are available.

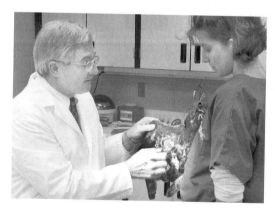

Many veterinary medical colleges offer exciting opportunities for students wishing to pursue a career in wildlife preservation. Here, a student assists in the examination of an injured red-tailed hawk at the Southeastern Raptor Rehabilitation Center at Auburn University's College of Veterinary Medicine.

Virginia-Maryland Regional College of Veterinary Medicine

Admissions Coordinator
Virginia-Maryland Regional College of Veterinary Medicine
Blacksburg VA 24061
Telephone: (540) 231-4699
Fax: (540) 231-9290
Email: dvmadmit@vt.edu
www.vetmed.vt.edu

The Virginia-Maryland Regional College of Veterinary Medicine is situated on 3 distinct campuses. The main campus is at Virginia Tech in Blacksburg, Virginia, a community with a population of about 40,000 situated on a high plateau in southwestern Virginia between the Blue Ridge and Allegheny Mountains. Its residents enjoy a wide range of educational, social, recreational, and cultural opportunities. In addition to the Blacksburg campus, the Equine Medical Center campus is in Leesburg, Virginia, and the University of Maryland is at College Park. The college received full accreditation in 1993 from the American Veterinary Medical Association.

In recognition of a need for veterinarians trained in both basic and clinical sciences, the college offers students the opportunity to participate in graduate studies and receive appropriate advanced training to conduct research in basic or clinical disciplines. Nearly 25 percent of the nation's veterinarians work in areas other than private practice, such as government and corporate veterinary medicine. Through the assistance of a grant from the Pew Charitable Trusts, the college has established the Center for Government and Corporate Veterinary Medicine, which is a national resource for training veterinarians for the wide variety of careers in this area of the profession.

Application Information

For specific application information (availability, deadlines, fees, and VMCAS participation), please refer to the contact information listed above.

Residency implications: 50 positions are reserved for Virginia residents, and 30 positions for Maryland residents. Up to 10 additional positions may be filled by nonresidents. Priority for nonresident positions will be given to residents of states without an accredited state-supported veterinary school.

Prerequisites for Admission

Course requirements and semester hours

Biological sciences (with laboratories)	8
Organic chemistry (with laboratories)	8
Physics (with laboratories)	8
Biochemistry	3
English (composition, 3 credit hours)	6
Humanities/social science	6
Mathematics (algebra, geometry, trigonometry, calculus)	6

Students must earn a C– or better in all required courses.

Science courses taken 7 or more years ago may be repeated or substituted with higher-level courses with the written consent of the admissions committee.

Required undergraduate GPA: to be considered for admission, applicants must have a cumulative GPA of at least 2.80 on a 4.00 scale upon completion of a minimum of 2 academic years of full-time study (60 semester/90 quarter hours) at an accredited college or university. Alternatively, a 3.30 GPA in the last 2 years (60 semester hours) will qualify a student who does not have a 2.80 GPA overall. All courses taken during this 2-year period must be junior or senior level. The mean GPA of those accepted into the class of 2009 was 3.50.

Advanced placement credit for 1 semester of English will be accepted if the additional required hours are composition or technical writing and are taken at a college or university.

Advanced placement credit or credit by examination for preveterinary course requirements will be accepted. Those credits must appear on the applicant's college transcript. Advanced placement credits will not be calculated in grade point averages and no grade assigned. No course substitutions will be allowed for AP credit or credit by examination.

Course completion deadline: required courses must be completed by the end of the spring term of the year in which matriculation occurs.

Standardized examinations: Graduate Record Examination (GRE®) is required. The GRE must have been taken after October 1, 2002.

Additional requirements and considerations

Maturity and a broad cultural perspective
Motivation and dedication to a career in veterinary medicine

Evidence of potential, and appreciation of the career opportunities for veterinarians, as indicated by:

1. Clinical veterinary experience (private practice)
2. Animal experience in addition to time spent working with a veterinarian
3. Veterinary experience outside of private clinical practice, such as research, industrial, government, and corporate settings
4. Extramural activities, achievements, honors
5. Communication skills
6. References

Summary of Admission Procedure

Timetable

Application deadline: October 2
Date interviews are held: February
Date acceptances mailed: early March
School begins: mid-August

Deposit (to hold place in class): $450.00 for Maryland and Virginia residents; $1,000.00 for nonresidents.

Deferments: case-by-case basis if a candidate has extenuating circumstances beyond his or her control.

Evaluation criteria

The admission procedure is comprised of an initial screening of applicants, an interview of selected applicants, and a final review of the dossiers of all interviewees.

	% weight
Academics	50
Cumulative GPA, required science GPA, last 45 semester-hour GPA, GRE® aptitude	
Background	25
Related animal experience; veterinary experience; research, industrial, and commercial experience; activities, achievements, and awards; narrative and personal references	
Interviews	25

2005–2006 admissions summary

	Number of Applicants	Number of New Entrants
Resident		
Maryland	78	30
Virginia	151	50
Nonresident	556	10
Total:	785	90

Expenses for the 2005–2006 Academic Year

Tuition and fees

Resident	$13,769.00
Nonresident	$30,969.00

Dual-Degree Programs

Combined DVM–graduate degree programs are available.

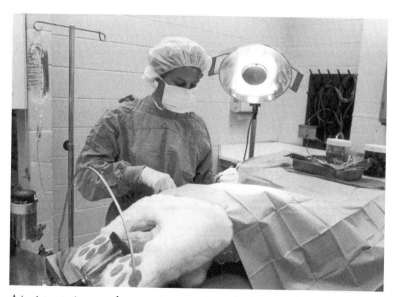

A junior veterinary student practices suturing techniques during the "Teddy Bear Repair Clinic" at the Virginia-Maryland Regional College of Veterinary Medicine's annual Open House. Photo courtesy of Biomedical Media Center, VMRCVM.

Washington State University

Office of Student Services
College of Veterinary Medicine
Washington State University
P. O. Box 647012
Pullman WA 99164-7012
Telephone: (509) 335-1532

Washington State University, which has an enrollment of 16,516, is located in southeastern Washington in the town of Pullman. This small community is surrounded by farmland yet is close to the mountains of Idaho. The area offers excellent summer and winter recreation.

The College of Veterinary Medicine at WSU was founded in 1899 and is one of the 5 oldest colleges of veterinary medicine in the country. Washington and Idaho have developed a regional program in veterinary medical education that also serves Arizona, Hawaii, Montana, Nevada, New Mexico, North Dakota, Utah, and Wyoming through the Western Interstate Commission for Higher Education (WICHE) Compact.

Upon satisfactory completion of this program, the Doctor of Veterinary Medicine (DVM) degree is conferred by the Regents of Washington State University. While the University of Idaho is a full partner in the program, Idaho students actually receive their DVM degrees from WSU.

Application Information

For specific application information (availability, deadlines, fees, and VMCAS participation), please refer to the contact information listed above.

Residency implications: in general, first preference is given to qualified applicants who are residents of Washington or Idaho, as well as qualified applicants certified by WICHE contract states. Second preference is given to qualified applicants from non-service area states and non-certified applicants from WICHE states.

Prerequisites for Admission

Course requirements

Biological Science:	(8 semester hours w/laboratory) The biology of organisms; plants, animals ecology, and evolution, including cellular and molecular biology and genetics. (WSU Biol 106 & 107)
Inorganic Chemistry:	(8 semester hours w/laboratory) Stoichiometry, structure, gases, liquids, solids, solutions, thermodynamics, kinetics, equilibrium, volumetric and gravimetric analysis. Acid-base, ionic, molecular, solubility, oxidation/reduction equilibria, kinetics, electro-chemistry, systematic chemistry of the elements, coordination compounds. (WSU Chem 105 & 106)
Organic Chemistry:	(4–5 semester hours w/laboratory) Structure and function in organic chemistry; reaction mechanisms, molecular orbital theory, alkanes, alkenes, alkynes, and radicals; biological applications. (WSU Chem 345)
Biochemistry:	(3 semester hours upper division) Proteins (amino acids, protein structure, enzyme kinetics and mechanisms); Metabolism (carbohydrate structure, glycolysis, TCA cycle, oxidative phosphorylation, glycogen metabolism, and metabolic integration); Molecular genetics (Central dogma, DNA structure, packaging, replication, repair, RNA transcription, translation, genetic code, protein targeting, gene expression, DNA technology). (WSU MBioS 303)
Mathematics:	(3 semester hours) Elementary functions; graphs, properties, and applications of polynomial, rational, exponential, logarithmic, and trigonometric functions. (WSU Math 107 or equivalent*)

Physics:	(4 credit hrs or 2 qtr) Algebra/trigonometry-based physics; topics in mechanics, wave phenomena, temperature, and heat. (WSU Phys 101)
Genetics:	(4 semester hours upper division) Basic mendelian genetics, meisosis, mitosis, chromosome rearrangement, DNA structure and replication, mutations, bacterial and phage genetics, gene regulation, transcription, translation, plasmids, transposons, cloning, population genetics, evolution. (WSU MBioS 301)
Statistics:	(3 semester hours) Graphical methods, descriptive statistics, measures of central tendency, probability distributions, variables, estimates and sample sizes, hypothesis testing, inferences, experimental design, and randomization) (WSU Stat 212)

*This course is recommended preparation for chemistry and physics courses. It will not satisfy the mathematics general education requirement, which calls for a calculus-based course or statistical thinking course.

Total minimum number of credits required is 60 semester hours or 90 quarter hours.

Required undergraduate GPA: none; a minimum overall GPA of 3.20 on a 4.00 scale is recommended. The class of 2009 had a mean overall GPA of 3.60 at the time of acceptance.

AP credit policy: to be reviewed.

Course completion deadline: prerequisite courses must be completed by June 15 prior to entry.

Standardized examinations: Graduate Record Examination (GRE®), general test, is required. Test scores older than 5 years will not be accepted. The mean combined score on the Graduate Record Examination for the class of 2009 was at the 58th percentile.

Additional requirements and considerations

Animal/veterinary work experience
Recommendations (3 required, one by a veterinarian)
Extracurricular and/or community service activities

Summary of Admission Procedure

Timetable

    Application deadline: October 2
    Date interviews are held: late February–early March
    Date acceptances mailed: March–April
    School begins: late August

Deposit (to hold place in class): none required

Deferments: are considered for financial reasons and completion of graduate degrees.

Evaluation criteria

Applicants will be selected based upon ability to successfully complete the program and demonstration of the qualities of a good veterinarian. Academic criteria include undergraduate, science, GRE test scores, and rigor of academic program (and quality of graduate program, if applicable). Nonacademic factors include maturity, integrity, compassion, communication skills, and desire to contribute to society. An interview will be required for residents of Washington, Idaho, and out-of-area applicants. WICHE applicants are ranked for WICHE funding using the same criteria above minus the interview.

2005–2006 admissions summary

	Number of Applicants	Number of New Entrants
Washington	115	59
Idaho	34	11
WICHE†	205	19
Arizona	63	2
Hawaii	15	1
Montana	20	6
Nevada	17	3
New Mexico	32	1
North Dakota	9	0
Utah	32	5
Wyoming	17	1
Nonresident	434	18
Total:	788	106

† For further information, see the listing of contracting states and provinces.

Expenses for the 2005–2006 Academic Year

Tuition and fees

Resident (WA, ID, and WICHE certified)	$13,776.00
Nonresident	$34,004.00

Western University of Health Sciences

Office of Admission
College of Veterinary Medicine
Western University of Health Sciences
309 East 2nd Street
Pomona, CA 91766-1854
Phone: (909) 623-6116
FAX: (909) 469-5570
E-mail: admissions@westernu.edu
Web site: http://www.western.edu/admissions/dvm_requirements.htm

Western University of Health Sciences is an independent, accredited, non-profit university incorporated in the State of California, dedicated to educating compassionate and scientifically competent health professionals who value diversity and a humanistic approach to patient care. The university, located in the San Gabriel Valley of Southern California, about 30 miles east of Los Angeles, grants postbaccalaureate professional degrees in five colleges: the College of Allied Health Professions, the College of Graduate Nursing, the College of Osteopathic Medicine of the Pacific, the College of Pharmacy, and the College of Veterinary Medicine. The College of Veterinary Medicine has been approved for the first steps of the accreditation process and admitted its first class in the fall of 2003. The founding principles of the College of Veterinary Medicine include:

1) *Commitment to student-centered, life-long learning.*
   The curriculum is designed to teach students to find and critically evaluate information, to enhance student cooperative learning, and to provide an environment for professional development.

2) *Commitment to a Reverence for Life philosophy in teaching veterinary medicine.*
   The College strives to make the educational experience one that enhances moral development of its students and is respectful to all animals and people involved in its programs.

3) *Commitment to excellence of student education through strategic partnerships in the public and private veterinary sectors.*
   This commitment seeks to maximize the learning experience in veterinary clinical practice and to educate practice-ready veterinarians capable of functioning independently upon graduation.

Phase I (Years 1 & 2): Basic and clinical veterinary science education using problem-based learning modules, a veterinary issues seminar series, a molecular biology seminar series, and an experiential clinical skills course.

Phase II (Year 3): Required rotations in thirteen different areas of veterinary medicine in regional veterinary practices or institutions including some rotations conducted on campus.

Phase III (Year 4): Selective rotations in regional, national or international specialty practices, veterinary teaching hospitals, or public/private institutions to be determined by students' career goals.

Application Information

For specific application information (availability, deadlines, fees, and VMCAS participation), please refer to the contact information listed previously.

Residency implications: applicants from all states as well as international applicants will be considered. In-state and out-of-state applicants are given *equal* consideration.

Prerequisites for Admissions

Course requirements:

	Semester Units	Quarter Units
Organic chemistry (including laboratory)	3	4
Biochemistry[2,3]	3	4
Biological & Life Sciences[4]	9	12
(including two upper division courses and one upper-division laboratory course)[3,5*]		
Microbiology[3,5]	3	4
Nutrition[3,5]	3	4
Genetics[3,5]	3	4
General physics (including laboratory)	6	8
Statistics[2]	3	4
English composition	3	4
Written communication in science or technology	3	4
Oral Communication	3	4
Psychology or sociology	3	4
Humanities/social sciences	6	8
Global Cultural/Financial Perspectives	3	4

*Ex: biology, physiology, anatomy, cell biology, embryology, zoology

1,2,3,4,5: See *Course completion deadline* on following page for details.

Required undergraduate GPA: Applicants must have a minimum overall GPA of 2.50 (undergraduate and graduate) at the time of application to be considered for admission. Prerequisite courses must be completed with a grade of C (or its equivalent) or higher.

AP credit policy: must appear on official college transcripts and be equivalent to the appropriate college-level coursework. AP test subject must also be specified on the transcript.

Course completion deadline: All courses must be completed at an accredited college or university in the U.S. or Canada *or* coursework completed outside the U.S. or Canada must be evaluated by a WesternU approved evaluation service.[1] Statistics course[2] must be a course designed or specified for science majors. Specified prerequisite courses[3] must have been completed no more than 8 years prior to the date of anticipated matriculation at WesternU-CVM. Classes taken after August 1, 1999, will be considered within the time limit and may be applied toward the prerequisites for the class entering Fall 2007. While not specifically required, courses in anatomy, physiology and embryology are strongly encouraged.[4] No more than two specified prerequisite courses[5] may be in progress after the end of the fall term immediately prior to matriculation. All required courses must be completed prior to matriculation. Failure to satisfactorily complete prerequisites with a grade of C or better will result in the loss of a candidate's seat in the class. One course cannot be used to satisfy more than one prerequisite.

Standardized examinations: Graduate Record Examination (GRE®), general test, or Medical College Admissions Test (MCAT) is required. Test scores must be submitted by the Ocober 16, 2006, deadline in the supplemental application packet. Test scores older than five years are not acceptable.

Additional requirements and considerations:

   Animal experience: must total at least 500 hours of hands-on experience that goes beyond observation. Appropriate venues include but are not limited to: animal medical environment/veterinary practice; commercial animal production; regulatory animal control; animal entertainment or research environment.

   Recommendations/evaluations: 3 are required from among the following: previous employers, supervisors of extended volunteer activities, academic personnel.
   Interview

Summary of Admissions Procedure

Timetable

    Primary application deadline: October 2
    Supplemental application deadline: October 16
    Date interviews are held: January–February
    Date acceptances mailed: March
    School begins: August

Deposit (to hold place in class): $500.

Deferments: request for deferments will be considered on a case-by-case basis.

Evaluation criteria:

    Academic achievement
    Standardized test performance
    Animal experience
    Letters of reference
    Interview
    Other supporting material

2005–2006 admissions summary

	Number of Applicants	Number of New Entrants
Resident	255	70
Nonresident	186	35
Total:	441	105

Expenses for the 2004–2005 Academic Year

Tuition and fees

Resident	$32,595.00
Nonresident	$32,595.00

University of Wisconsin

Office of Academic Affairs
School of Veterinary Medicine
2015 Linden Drive
University of Wisconsin-Madison
Madison WI 53706-1102
Telephone: (608) 263-2525
www.vetmed.wisc.edu.oaa

The University of Wisconsin is located in Madison, the state capital, which has a population of about 190,000. Consistently ranked among the nation's "most livable" cities, its hilly terrain, scattered parks, and woodlands saturate the urban setting with a friendly neighborhood atmosphere. Centered on a narrow isthmus among 4 scenic lakes, the city is a recreational paradise. The university sprawls over 900 acres along Lake Mendota and its student population is nearly 45,000. It has rated among the top 10 universities academically since 1910 and is third in the country in volume of research activity.

The School of Veterinary Medicine facility has a modern veterinary teaching hospital, modern equipment, and high-quality lab space for teaching and research. The curriculum provides a broad education in veterinary medicine with learning experiences in food animal medicine and other specialty areas. The school pioneered a unique senior rotation in ambulatory service for fourth-year students where they experience the life and work of a veterinarian specializing in large-animal medicine by working in one of 20 practices near Madison. The school has an outstanding research program with faculty in the forefront. Many faculty members have joint appointments with the College of Agriculture, the Medical School, the Regional Primate Center, the McArdle Cancer Research Institute, the National Wildlife Health Laboratory, and the North Central Dairy Forage Center. These outside links provide research and job opportunities for students.

Application Information

For specific application information (availability, deadlines, fees, and VMCAS participation), please refer to the contact information listed above.

Residency implications: between 60 and 70 Wisconsin residents will be accepted. Wisconsin has no contractual agreements, but may accept 10–20 nonresidents. Applicants who can claim legal residency or domicile in more than one state should contact the school. Wisconsin has a cooperative agreement with the Pontifical Catholic University of Puerto Rico and the

University of Puerto Rico-Mayaguez (UPR-Mayaguez) annually to offer admission to up to 2 students from the Pontifical Catholic University of Puerto Rico and UPR-Mayaguez. Students from Puerto Rico considering applying to the BS/DVM Binary Program should contact the College of Sciences, Pontifical Catholic University of Puerto Rico, Estacion 6, Ponce, Puerto Rico 00732 and/or the College of Agricultural Sciences, University of Puerto Rico-Mayaguez, P.O. Box 5000, Mayaguez, PR 00681-5000.

Prerequisites for Admission

Applicants must complete a minimum of 60 semester credits of college coursework. The 60 credits include the required 40–43 credits of coursework listed below, plus a minimum of 17 credits of elective coursework left to the student's discretion. The 17 elective credits allow the student to meet personal and academic goals and objectives while preparing for admission to veterinary school.

Course requirements and semester hours

General biology or zoology, introductory animal biology
    course (with laboratory)   5

General and qualitative chemistry, 2-semester lecture
    series (with laboratory)   8

Organic chemistry, 1-semester lecture satisfying bio-
    chemistry prerequisite   3

Biochemistry (organic chemistry must be prerequisite)   3

English composition or journalism   6

    Must include completion of either of the following:

    1. satisfactory score on a college English placement
       exam, or

    2. an introductory English composition course, plus
       completion of one of the following:

       a. an English composition or journalism course
          graded on the basis of writing skills, or

       b. written evidence from instructor that writing
          skills were included in the grading of a specific
          college-level course

Genetics or animal breeding, must include principles of
    heredity and preferably molecular mechanisms   3

General physics, 2-semester lecture series   6

Statistics, introductory course   3

Social sciences/humanities, any elective courses in so-
    cial science or the humanities   6

Required undergraduate GPA: the mean cumulative GPA of the class of 2009 is approximately 3.47 for residents and 3.49 for nonresidents.

AP credit policy: must appear on official college transcripts and be equivalent to the appropriate college-level coursework.

Course completion deadline: all coursework must be completed no later than the spring 2007 term prior to admission to the fall 2007 term.

Standardized examinations: Graduate Record Examination (GRE®), general test, is required. All applicants are required to take or retake the GRE, including the writing assessment. The GRE may be taken no later than October 2 in the year of application. The mean score of the class of 2009 for the verbal and quantitative portions combined is approximately 1213 for residents and 1235 for nonresidents.

Additional requirements and considerations

    Animal contact and work experience
    Veterinary medical experience
    Other preparatory experience
    College degrees earned
    Extracurricular activities
    Recommendations/evaluations (3 required)
    Scholarships/awards
    Diversity
    Personal statement

Summary of Admission Procedure

Timetable

    Application deadline: October 2
    Interviews: none
    Date acceptances mailed: mid-March
    School begins: early September

Deposit (to hold place in class): none required.

Deferments: are considered on an individual basis by the Admissions Committee and may be granted for extenuating circumstances.

Evaluation criteria

There is a 2-part admission procedure. For the fall 2005 admission year, the class was selected based upon the following comparative evaluation:

1. *Evaluation of academic record* (weighted approximately 60 percent)
    Undergraduate cumulative GPA
    Required course GPA
    Most recent 30 semester credit GPA
    GRE® test scores
2. *Evaluation of personal experience and characteristics*
   (weighted approximately 40 percent)
    Animal and veterinary work experience
    Other preparatory experience (includes extracurricular activities)
    Personal history/academic performance (summary category to include re-
       view of academic history, academic achievements, diversity of back-
       ground, etc.)
    Reference letters

2004–2005 admissions summary

	Number of Applicants	Number of New Entrants
Resident	168	60
Nonresident	704	20
Total:	872	80

Expenses for the 2004–2005 Academic Year

Tuition and fees
    Resident $15,843.00
    Nonresident $23,874.00

Dual-Degree Programs

Combined DVM–graduate degree programs are available.

INTERNATIONAL VETERINARY MEDICAL SCHOOLS

University of Edinburgh
Royal (Dick) School of Veterinary Studies

Undergraduate Admissions Officer
School Office
Royal (Dick) School of Veterinary Studies
The University of Edinburgh
Summerhall
Edinburgh EH9 1QH
Scotland, UK
Tel: +44 (0)131 6506178
Fax: +44 (0)131 6506585
Email: geraldine.giannopoulos@ed.ac.uk
http://www.vet.ed.ac.uk

The Royal (Dick) School of Veterinary Studies, established in 1823, was the first veterinary school in Scotland, and the second to be established in the UK. The long-standing involvement of Edinburgh with veterinary education, where tradition is mixed with cutting-edge veterinary teaching, benefits from a closely-knit collegial community of "Dick" vet students. As one of only 5 international vet schools with AVMA accreditation, the veterinary degree course at Edinburgh (BVM&S) provides an excellent foundation for a subsequent career in veterinary practice or one of the many related career opportunities, such as biomedical research. The academic and research environment in Edinburgh is internationally recognised for encouraging excellence in a broad base of teaching and learning. The school is on 2 sites: one in central Edinburgh and the other at the Easter Bush Veterinary Centre in nearby Roslin, approximately 10 kilometres south of the city. Our split site permits the benefits of an urban setting, while allowing us the luxury of space in the rural setting.

The city of Edinburgh, the capital of Scotland, is one of Europe's most handsome cities. The beauty of its setting and its architecture, allied with its intellectual traditions, have earned the title of "Athens of the North" for what is still a compact city of some 500,000 people. It is a city of noted buildings, fine gardens, and open spaces, including Holyrood Park—one of the largest city centre natural parks in Europe—and Princes Street Gardens, between the Old and New Towns. The city offers students a rich mix of academic, social and allied facilities—libraries, museums and art galleries, concert halls, theatres and cinemas. The city has easy access to coastline, lochs, mountains and countryside, with ready-made opportunities for open-air sports and recreation.

Further details on the BVM&S degree programme, the School and its facilities can be found by visiting http://www.vet.ed.ac.uk.

Application Information

For specific application information (availability, deadlines, fees and VMCAS participation), please refer to the contact information listed above.

Residency implications: US nationals entering the UK as students do not require a visa and are categorised as non-visa nationals. However, due to recent changes in immigration legislation students from the USA (who are planning to come to the UK for more than 6 months, after November 2003) are now required to obtain an entry clearance certificate prior to entering the UK. For further information on entry to the UK, please refer to http://www.ukvisas.gov.uk.

Students must also be able to ensure adequate financial support for the duration of their course.

Prerequisites for Admission

Course requirements

A minimum of at least 2 years of full-time study in a preveterinary or science course at college or university. A minimum of one year (2 semesters or 3 terms) in chemistry and biology with additional courses in physics and/or mathematics is required. All applicants are required to have gained high grades in the science subjects, especially chemistry.

A number of places are available in the graduate entry programme (GEP) for candidates who hold a suitable degree in biological sciences.

Required undergraduate GPA: 3.4 (on 4.0 point scale)

Course completion deadline: all required courses should be completed prior to August of the year of admission.

Additional requirements and considerations

Applicants are also expected to have gained relevant work experience of handling animals. This should, where possible, include not only seeing veterinary practice, but also spending time on livestock farms and other animal establishments.

Summary of Admission Procedure

Timetable

Application deadline: October 2
Date acceptances mailed: early April at the latest
Interviews: early–mid March (held in the U.S.)
School begins: mid-September or early August (for GEP entrants)

Deposit: After an offer has been made, a deposit of £1,500 is required by mid-May to hold a position in the class

Deferments: Not applicable

Evaluation criteria

Academic performance
Animal/veterinary experience
Personal statement
Motivation
References/Evaluations (minimum 2 required—one from academic science source and one from a veterinary surgeon)
Interview

2004–2005 admissions summary (for entry in 2005)*

	Number of Applicants	Number of New Entrants
In-province	1,140	100
International	200	20
Total	1,340	120

*The University of Edinburgh joined VMCAS in admissions cycle 2003–2004.

Expenses for the 2006–2007 Academic Year*

Tuition and fees

Resident	residents of the UK are government-funded
International	£16,550*

*for up-to-date information on fees and all further information regarding admission to the School, please visit our website.

University of Glasgow

Mrs. Joyce Wason
Director of Student Services
University of Glasgow Veterinary School
Bearsden Road
Bearsden Glasgow G61 1QH
Tel: (+44) 141 330 5705
Fax: (+44) 141 942 7215
Email: J.Wason@vet.gla.ac.uk

The Glasgow Veterinary College was founded in 1862 and incorporated into the University of Glasgow in 1949. Initially Veterinary Medicine was part of the Faculty of Medicine, but in 1968 the independent Faculty of Veterinary Medicine was formed. Now set in the grounds of a beautiful wooded estate, the Glasgow University Veterinary School has grown to become one of the largest in the UK, with an enviable record in teaching and research. Founded by Papal Bull in 1451, Glasgow University is the fourth-oldest university in Britain after Oxford, Cambridge, and St. Andrews. Throughout its history the focus of the university has been on excellence in teaching and research.

The city of Glasgow has a population of around 74,000 and is Scotland's largest city. One of Europe's liveliest places with a varied and colorful cultural and social life, it can cater to every taste. Situated on the River Clyde, Glasgow has excellent road and rail links to the rest of the UK and air services to a wide range of destinations, both home and overseas.

Application Information

For specific application information (availability, deadlines, fees, and VMCAS participation), please refer to the contact information listed above.

Residency implications: U.S. nationals entering the UK as students do not require a visa and are categorized as non-visa nationals. However, due to recent changes in immigration legislation, students from the U.S. (who are planning to come to the UK for more than 6 months) are now required to obtain an entry clearance certificate prior to entering the UK. For further information on entry to the UK, please refer to http://www.ukvisas.gov.uk. Students must also be able to ensure adequate financial support for the duration of their course.

Prerequisites for Admission

Course requirements

3 years of full-time university study; subjects to include organic chemistry, biology, math, and (if possible) a knowledge of physics and a cumulative average of around 70%.

Required undergraduate GPA: 3.40.

AP credit policy: not applicable.

Course completion deadline: required courses should be completed prior to admission in the fall.

Standardized examinations: none required. GRE® results will be considered if submitted.

Additional requirements and considerations

Animal/veterinary work experience sufficient to indicate motivation, interest, and understanding of the veterinary profession
Evaluations: minimum 2, one each from an academic science source and a veterinary surgeon.

Summary of Admission Procedure

Timetable

    Application deadline: October 3
    Date interviews held: February–March (in the U.S.)
    Date acceptances mailed: April
    School begins: late September
Deposit (to hold place in class): £1,000
Deferments: in certain circumstances.

Evaluation criteria

    Academic performance
    Animal/veterinary experience
    References
    Essay
    Interview

2003–2004 admissions summary

	Number of Applicants	Number of New Entrants
In-province	1,200	73
International	300	45
Total:	1,500	118

Expenses for the 2005–2006 Academic Year

Tuition and fees

Resident	residents of the UK are government-funded
International	£16,500

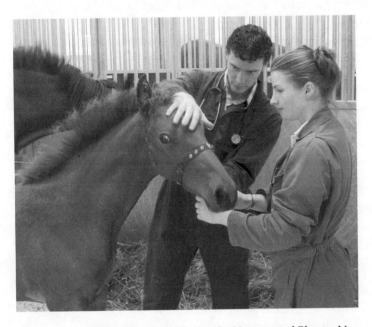

The Equine Centre for Equine Welfare at the University of Glasgow Veterinary School offers state-of-the-art technology to children's ponies and to Cheltenham winners alike. Photo courtesy of Joyce Wason, University of Glasgow Veterinary School.

University of Guelph

Admissions, Office of Registrarial Services
University Centre, Level 3
University of Guelph
Guelph Ontario N1G 2W1
Canada
Telephone: (519) 824-4120, ext. 56062
www.ovc.uoguelph.ca

Founded in 1862, the Ontario Veterinary College is located in Guelph about 60 miles north of Buffalo. Guelph has a similar climate to Detroit and Chicago. Surrounded by gently rolling farmland, this city of 100,000 is typical of the northeast.

The university has an enrollment of 15,000 undergraduate students, of whom 440 are veterinary students. There are also approximately 150 graduate students, 100 faculty, and 200 staff members at the veterinary college, which offers degree programs leading to a DVM, MS, PhD, Doctor of Veterinary Science (DVSc) and a Graduate Diploma. The college has 4 departments—Population Medicine, Clinical Studies, Biomedical Sciences, and Pathobiology—and a full-service teaching hospital. Funding for research comes from 2 sources: the Ontario Ministry of Agriculture, Food and Rural Affairs research contract of 4.6 million \$C and external research grants and contracts of 3.9 million \$C. There are also large, modern research stations for separately housing sheep, swine, and dairy and beef cattle.

Application Information

For specific application information (availability, deadlines, fees, and VMCAS participation), please refer to the contact information listed above.

Residency implications: International applicants will be considered provided the applicant does not hold Canadian citizenship or permanent resident status in Canada. There is a maximum of 5 international positions available per year.

Prerequisites for Admission

Course requirements and semester hours: Students must first complete a minimum of two full-time years (four full-time semesters) of university including specific university courses. Students initially apply for admission to a science degree program. For the purpose of DVM admission, a full-time semester will include at least 5 one-semester courses. Once the prerequisite courses are completed successfully, students apply for admission to the DVM Program. The subject matter requirements listed below must have been completed before admission to the DVM program will be considered.

Course requirements and semesters

Biological sciences (emphasis on animal biology; one semester must be cell biology)	3
Genetics	1
Biochemistry	1
Statistics (with a university-level calculus prerequisite)	1
Humanities or social sciences*	2

* Students entering the DVM program should be able to operate across discipline boundaries recognizing the relevance of the humanities and social sciences to their career choice. In selecting these courses from among those acceptable, the prospective veterinary student should consider topics such as ethics, logic, critical thinking, determinants of human behavior, and human social interaction.

Required courses proposed to be completed at an institution other than the University of Guelph should be approved as acceptable prior to registration. Applicants are required to request approval for courses in writing. Course descriptions *must* be included with the request. Courses will *not* be acceptable if they are repeats of previously passed courses, or if they are taken at the same or a lower level in a subject area than previously passed courses in the same subject area. It is expected that the required undergraduate preparation for the DVM program will be completed in a full-time coherent academic program.

Required undergraduate GPA: students with a minimum GPA of 3.00 on a 4.00 scale based on the average of the required courses and the last 2 semesters in full-time attendance at university may be further considered.

Course completion deadline: required courses must be completed by June 15 of the year of application in order to be further considered.

Standardized examinations: Medical College Admission Test (MCAT) is required. Test scores must be received no later than December 1 of the year of application. (Applicants may submit GRE® scores in lieu of MCAT scores.)

Additional requirements and considerations

Reasons for choosing a career in veterinary medicine

Quality of preparatory academic program

Experience and knowledge in matters relating to animals and to the veterinary medical profession

Experience and achievement in extracurricular affairs and/or community
service activities
Communication skills
Referees' reports

Summary of Admission Procedure

Timetable

Application deadline: October 2 for VMCAS applications; December 1
for all others
Date interviews are held: February–June
Date acceptances mailed: March–July
School begins: September
Deposit (to hold place in class): $500.00

2005–2006 admissions summary

	Number of Applicants	Number of New Entrants
Residents	350	105
International Residents	100	5
Total:	450	110

Expenses for the 2005–2006 Academic Year

Tuition and fees

Resident	$5,500.00 $C
Visa student	$44,500.00 $C

Massey University

International Student Affairs
Massey University Veterinary School
Institute of Veterinary, Animal and Biomedical Sciences
College of Sciences
Massey University
Private Bag 11-222
Palmerston North
New Zealand
Tel: (+64) 6350 4473
Fax (+64) 6350 5699
Email: vetschool@massey.ac.nz
http://vet-school.massey.ac.nz/

Massey University is located "down under" in picturesque New Zealand. The vet school is located in Palmerston North, a student-friendly town of 75,000 in the lower central north island of New Zealand. Nicknamed "student city," Palmerston North offers free bus service and free bikes to Massey students and is home to numerous cafés, restaurants, bars, theatres, and outdoor recreational activities. Palmerston North is a one-hour flight from Auckland and just under a two-hour drive to Wellington City and the ski fields of Mt. Ruapehu.

The Massey University Veterinary School accepts up to 24 international students annually with a total class size of just less than 100. The first class of Massey veterinarians graduated in 1967, and since then more than 2,500 veterinarians have graduated and are working around the world.

The Massey University veterinary degree has an international reputation for providing an excellent veterinary education with a strong science background, a broad knowledge of companion, equine, and production animal health, and a focus on independent thinking and problem-solving skills. The curriculum incorporates practical aspects throughout all years of the degree beginning with animal handling and behaviour in the first post-selection semester through to the final year of the program, which is almost entirely clinically based.

The veterinary facilities are of a high international standard with numerous other university-run animal units (farms, equine blood typing unit, feline unit, large animal teaching unit, etc.) on or adjacent to the Palmerston North campus. The veterinary teaching hospital sees first-opinion cases as well as referral cases to provide a balanced clinical experience for the students. The staff at the Massey University Veterinary School are collegial, motivated, highly qualified individuals, many of whom have trained in the United States or are board-certified specialists in their discipline.

Studying abroad in New Zealand will give you the opportunity to see some of the world while studying toward your veterinary qualification and broadening your horizons and perspectives in life.

Application Information

For specific information (availability, deadlines, fees, and VMCAS participation), please refer to the contact information listed above.

Residency implications: All non-NZ students require a student visa, which is easily obtained following an offer of admission into the programme. Students must be able to ensure adequate financial support for the duration of their course.

Prerequisites for Admissions

Course requirements

Group 1—Competitive Selection into Vet School via Semester 1 (8 places available)
Group 1 applicants are required to come to Massey University and complete a pre-selection semester (beginning in late February of each year) of full-time study (4 classes) at Massey University in order to develop a GPA for selection.

Applicants need to meet eligibility requirements for admission to Massey University. Credit will be given where similar classes to the four pre-selection semester classes have already been completed, and other classes will be taken in their place.

Group 2—Competitive Selection directly into BVSc Semester 2 (16 places available)
Applicants are required to have completed two full years of full-time university education. Applicants need to have completed and passed classes equivalent to the 4 standard Massey University pre-veterinary semester classes:

Massey University Class	Usual classes needed for credit
Chemistry and Living Systems	• General chemistry • Organic chemistry
Physics for Life Sciences	• 1 year of physics
Biology of Cells	• Cell (molecular) biology • +/– Genetics
Biology of Animals	• Animal biology/zoology

Each of these classes should include laboratories.

Required undergraduate GPA: a minimum science GPA of 3.00 is required to be eligible to apply for the vet program.

Course completion deadline:

Group 2: all required courses should be completed by February 28 in the year of application.

Group 1: not applicable; courses completed in New Zealand.

Standardized examinations: Graduate Record Examination (GRE®), general test, is required for Group 2 applicants only. The minimum GRE score required is 1600 (this may be subject to change). Test scores can be no older than 5 years immediately preceding the application deadline. Score must be received by February 28 in the year of application.

Additional requirements and considerations:
A letter signed by a veterinarian on his/her clinic letterhead verifying that a minimum of 5 days of work experience at the clinic has been completed by the applicant.

Summary of Admission Procedure

Timetable

Group 1 (semester 1)
Application deadline: December 1
Date letters of admission to semester 1 sent: once completed application received
School begins: late February (semester 1)
Date acceptances into the vet program mailed: early July
Date vet program begins: mid-July (semester 2)

Group 2
Application deadline: February 28
Date acceptances mailed: mid-March
School begins: mid-July (semester 2)

Deposit (to hold Group 2 position): none required

Deferments: not applicable

Evaluation criteria

Group 1
Weighted GPA   80%
Minimum of a B average across all 4 first-semester classes needed to be eligible for selection.
Special Tertiary Admissions Test (STAT)   20%
This is the Australian equivalent to the GRE® and is held at Massey University at the end of the first semester.
Top 8 applicants offered places

Group 2
    Science GPA   50%
    GRE® General Test   50%
Top 16 applicants offered places

2005 admissions summary

	Number of Applicants	Number of New Entrants
Residents	276	82
International		
Group 1	26	5
Group 2	<u>30</u>	<u>12</u>
Total:	332	99

Expenses for the 2006 Academic Year

Tuition and fees

Resident	residents of New Zealand are government-subsidised

International   Semester 1 $NZ 9,000

Semesters 2–9 $NZ 20,000 ($NZ 40,000 per year)

The tuition fee in $US will depend on the current exchange rate at the time of payment. In 2006 the tuition fees were approximately $US 27,000.

Université de Montréal

Service des Admissions
Université de Montréal
C.P. 6205
Succursale Centre-Ville
Montréal Québec H3C 3T5
Canada
Téléphone: (514) 343-7076
Email: saefmv@medvet.umontreal.ca
www.medvet.umontreal.ca

Renseignements pour les applications/Application Information

Formulaires disponibles dès: décembre
Applications available: December

Date limite de remise: 1er mars
Application deadline: March 1

Frais d'application: 30.00 $C
Application fee: 30.00 $C

Statut de résident: Il faut être citoyen Canadien ou résident permanent pour
être admissible.
Residency implications: Canadian citizenship or permanent residency in Canada
is required.

Prérequis/Prerequisites for Admission

DEC (Diplôme d'Etudes Collégiales) en sciences de la nature
DEC (Junior College Diploma: obtained in Quebec) majoring in
nature science. (The DEC represents 2 years of post-high school
studies.)

Cours/Course requirements

Physique/Physics	101, 201, 301–78
Chimie/Chemistry	101, 201, 202
Biologie/Biology	301, 401
Mathématiques (avec calcul intégral)/	103, 203
Mathematics (including calculus)	

Pour être admis au programme de DMV, il faut: a) avoir satisfait les conditions ci-dessus, ou b) faire preuve d'études équivalentes.

To be considered for admission, one must: a) have completed the above requirements, or b) have completed equivalent studies.

Note: All lectures are given in French. Examinations must be written in French.

Le programme de DMV est maintenant réparti sur cinq ans.
The DMV is now a 5-year program.

La Maîtrise de la langue française est une condition de diplômation. Par conséquent, tout nouvel étudiant doit réussir le test de français du Ministère de l'Education ou, s'il échoue au test, réussir les cours de français prescrits par l'Université.

Test de Français: toute personne dont les deux dernières sessions d'études n'ont pas été faites en français doit subir un test de connaissance du français et obtenir un résultat égal ou supérieur à 83% avant de pouvoir s'inscrire au programme.

French test: All applicants who did not study language for the last two semesters of their studies must take a test to evaluate their knowledge of French. A passing grade of 83% is required to be admitted to the program.

Performance Score: This score is obtained by comparing the student's grade in each course with the class average.

Dossier academique avant admission: Le candidat doit, ou bien avoir terminé, ou s'être inscrit à tous les cours prérequis au moment de l'application.

Course completion deadline: The applicant must be registered for or have completed all prerequisites at the time of application.

Critères de sélection (priorité d'importance)/Additional considerations
(in order of importance)
  1. Dossier académique
  2. Entrevue: l'entrevue a été structurée pour évaluer la motivation, la préparation et le raisonnement des candidats.
  1. Academic record
  2. Interview: the interview is designed to verify the applicant's motivation, preparation, judgment, etc. The above list reflects priorities (applicants are judged first on academic merit, then test/exam results, etc.).

Cédule du processus/Summary of Admission Procedure

Horaire

Date limite de remise des formules: le 1er mars
Entrevues: mi-mai
Notification d'acceptation: fin mai, début juin
Début de l'année scolaire: fin août

Timetable

Application deadline: March 1
Interviews: mid-May
Notification of acceptance: end of May, early June
Fall semester begins: end of August

Dépôt nécessaire pour garder une place dans la classe: aucun.
Deposit (to hold place in class): none required.

L'acceptation ne peut, en aucun cas, être reportée à une année subséquente.
Deferments: not considered.

Critères d'évaluation/Evaluation criteria	%
Résultats scolaires/Performance score	60
Entrevue/Interview	40

Budget estimé/Estimated Expenses for the 2002–2003 Academic Year

Frais de scolarité: 55.61$C   par crédit pour les étudiants québécois (approx. 50 crédits par année)

Tuition and fees: 55.61 $C   per credit for residents of Quebec (approx. 50 per year)

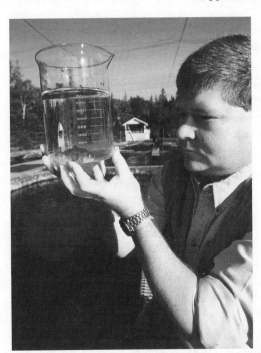

Fish health and aquaculture are expanding fields at some veterinary medical colleges. Photo courtesy of Atlantic Veterinary College, University of Prince Edward Island.

University of Prince Edward Island

Registrar's Office
Atlantic Veterinary College
University of Prince Edward Island
550 University Avenue
Charlottetown PEI C1A 4P3
Canada
Telephone: (902) 566-0608
Email: registrar@upei.ca
www.upei.ca/registrar/

The Atlantic Veterinary College (AVC), one of the newest colleges of veterinary medicine in North America, opened in 1986 and is fully accredited by the American Veterinary Medical Association, the Canadian Veterinary Medical Association, and the Royal College of Veterinary Surgeons (UK).

Centrally located on Canada's eastern seaboard (650 miles northeast of Boston), the Atlantic Veterinary College makes its home in a beautiful island setting in Charlottetown, Prince Edward Island. With a population of 138,000, which jumps to over a million during the summer tourist season, the community enjoys a small-town lifestyle that boasts the amenities of larger cities, including dining and theatre. Residents also enjoy outdoor activities, such as golfing, cycling, sailing, and cross-country skiing.

The college is a completely integrated teaching, research, and service facility. The four-story complex contains the veterinary teaching hospital, diagnostic services, fish health unit, farm services, postmortem services, animal barns, laboratories, classrooms, computer and audio-visual facilities, offices, cafeteria, and study areas. The Atlantic Veterinary College also operates a nearby farm facility, a swine research facility, and a fish hatchery.

Prince Edward Island is a scenic province with a wide variety of dairy, beef, hog, sheep, horse, and fish farms. The combination and variety of animal and fish farms have allowed AVC to develop a special expertise in fish health, aquaculture, and population medicine.

Application Information

For specific application information (availability, deadlines, fees, and VMCAS participation), please refer to the contact information listed above.

Residency implications: Atlantic Veterinary College contracts with New Brunswick (13), Newfoundland (2), Nova Scotia (11), and the home province P.E.I. (10). International students are admitted on a noncontract basis (24).

Prerequisites for Admission

The preveterinary program leading to admission at the Atlantic Veterinary College will normally be completed within the context of a 2-year science program.

Course requirements

Twenty-one semester courses or equivalent are required. Normally, these courses must be completed while the applicant is enrolled as a full-time student carrying at least 15 semester hours' credit. Science courses will normally have a laboratory component and be completed within 6 years of the date of application. Exceptional circumstances will be given consideration; however, it is necessary for all applicants to demonstrate the ability to master difficult subject matter in the context of meaningful full-time activity.

Courses must include:

Mathematics	1 course
Statistics	1 course
Biological sciences	2 courses, with an emphasis on animal biology* with labs
Microbiology	1 course with lab
Genetics	1 course
Chemistry	3 courses, including organic chemistry with labs
Physics	1 course with lab
English	2 courses, including 1 course in English composition
Humanities and social sciences	3 courses
Electives	5 courses from any discipline

* Examples of animal biology courses include first-year general biology, vertebrate anatomy, vertebrate histology, vertebrate physiology, vertebrate zoology, molecular biology, and cell biology.

It is recommended that applicants consider including courses in the following topics in their preveterinary curriculum: personal finance, small business management, psychology, sociology, biochemistry, ethics, and logic.

Required undergraduate GPA: no minimum stated; mean cumulative GPA of most recent entering class is 3.20 on a 4.00 scale.

AP credit policy: not accepted.

Course completion deadline: June 1 of the year of application.

Standardized examinations: Graduate Record Examination (GRE®) (for non-Canadian applicants only). If a student's native language or language of prior education is not English, then the student will be required to pass one of the following: TOEFL, MELAB, IELB, or CanTest.

Additional requirements and considerations

Veterinary-related experience: at least two 40-hour experiences with veterinarians in practice, government, industry, or in a research environment at an academic institution are required. One of these experiences must involve clinical practice in the field. If an applicant selects 2 clinical experiences, these 2 experiences cannot be in the same field—e.g., large, small, exotics—or take place under the supervision of the same veterinarian.

Veterinary evaluations: immediate family members cannot complete evaluation.

Interview

Essay

Summary of Admission Procedure

Timetable

Application deadline: October 2 for VMCAS applications; November 1 for supplementary application; and January 1 for transfer

Date interviews are held: February–March

Date acceptances mailed: April

School begins: late August; registration, early September

Deposit (to hold place in class): 500.00 $C

Deferments: are considered for extenuating circumstances.

Evaluation criteria

Academic credentials and animal work experience are objectively evaluated by the Registrar's Office. Other criteria and activities are evaluated by the admissions committee through an interview process.

	% weight
Grades	55
Veterinary experience, interview	35
Essay	10

2004–2005 admissions summary

	Number of Applicants	Number of New Entrants
In-province	24	10
Contract*	90	26
International	190	24
Total:	304	60

Expenses for the 2003–2004 Academic Year

Tuition and fees

Resident	7,990.00 $C
Contract student*	7,990.00 $C
International student	45,110.00 $C

* For further information, see the listing of contracting states and provinces.

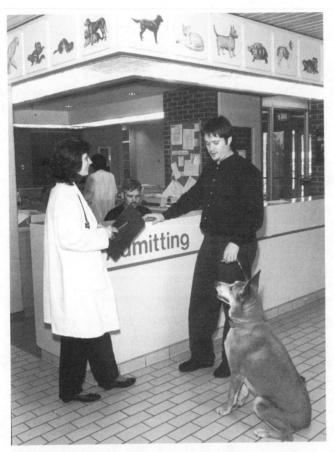

Small-animal care in a clinic is but one of many options for hands-on training at veterinary medical colleges. Photo courtesy of Atlantic Veterinary College, University of Prince Edward Island.

University of Saskatchewan

Admissions Office
Western College of Veterinary Medicine
52 Campus Drive
University of Saskatchewan
Saskatoon Saskatchewan S7N 5B4
Canada
Telephone: (306) 966-7454
www.usask.ca/wcvm

The Western College of Veterinary Medicine is located in the city of Saskatoon, which has a population of about 220,000 and is the major urban center in central Saskatchewan. The city is also the major commercial center for central and northern Saskatchewan and is served by 2 national airlines with direct connections to all major centers in Canada.

The Western College of Veterinary Medicine is one of the few veterinary colleges where all health sciences and agriculture are offered on the same campus. The college is devoted to undergraduate education and has a reputation in Canada and in the northwestern United States for educating veterinarians who are well-rounded in general veterinary medicine and have good practical backgrounds. It has one of the best field-service caseloads in North America.

Application Information

For specific application information (availability, deadlines, fees, and VMCAS participation), please refer to the contact information listed above.

Residency implications: students are selected for quota positions from Alberta, British Columbia, Manitoba, Saskatchewan, and the Yukon, Nunavut, and Northwest Territories. Special consideration is given to self-identified individuals of aboriginal origin. Residents of foreign countries are not considered.

Prerequisites for Admission

Course requirements and semester hours

English	6
Physics	6
Biology	6
Genetics	3
Introductory chemistry	6
Organic chemistry	3
Mathematics or statistics	6
Biochemistry	6
Microbiology	3
Electives	15

Required undergraduate GPA: a minimum cumulative average of 70% is required.

Course completion deadline: prerequisite courses must be completed by the time of entry into the program.

Standardized examinations: none required.

Additional requirements and considerations

Animal/veterinary work experience, motivation, and knowledge
Maturity
Leadership
Communication skills

Summary of Admission Procedure

Timetable

Application deadline: January 3
Date interviews are held: May–June
Date acceptances mailed: on or before July 1
School begins: late August
Deposit (to hold place in class): none required.
Deferments: not considered.

Evaluation criteria

The 3-part admission procedure consists of an assessment of academic ability, a personal interview, and an overall assessment of the application file.

	% weight
Grades	60
Interview*	30
Judgement	10

* Interview selection is based entirely on academic performance.

2005–2006 admissions summary

	Number of Applicants	Number of New Entrants
Resident	65	21
Contract†	222	50
Nonresident	1	0
Total:	288	71

Expenses for the 2005–2006 Academic Year

Tuition and fees

Resident	7,001.00 $C
Nonresident	
Contract student†	7,001.00 $C
Other nonresident-Canadian	7,001.00 $C

† For further information, see the listing of contracting states and provinces.

POLICIES ON ADVANCED STANDING

Transfers are permitted to most colleges of veterinary medicine in the United States under specified conditions. Typical requirements include a vacancy in the class, completion of all prerequisite requirements, and compatible curricula. Following is a listing of schools and some of the conditions under which they will consider a transfer from another veterinary college with advanced standing. More detailed information may be obtained by writing to the individual schools in which you have an interest.

UNITED STATES

Colorado State University

Advanced standing will be considered on an individual basis subject to the following provisions:

1. An open position must be available within the applicable tuition classification category for an additional student.
2. The applicant must meet all prerequisites for admission to the program as a first-year student and possess qualifications that are competitive with currently enrolled students.
3. The applicant must have completed at least one full academic year at the institution in which currently enrolled and have achieved a cumulative GPA of 3.00 or better (of 4.00) and be in good academic standing. Transfer credit will not be allowed for any course receiving a grade of less than 2.00 (of 4.00).
4. If the applicant is acceptable to the Admissions Committee and a position is available, placement will be offered in the year and term of the curriculum deemed appropriate after analysis of equivalency of the required courses.
5. Applicant must be enrolled in an AVMA accredited college.
6. Application deadlines: November 1 and April 1

Transfer students attending non-AVMA accredited institutions must apply for admission to the first-year class through the regular admissions process.

University of Florida

1. An opening must exist in the second- or third-year class.
2. Students are only rarely considered for advanced standing based on exceptional personal circumstances.
3. Student must be enrolled in an AVMA accredited college.

4. Student must meet all prerequisites for admission as a first-year student (including GRE® scores).
5. The curricula of the two schools must be sufficiently alike to allow a student to enter without deficiencies in academic background.
6. Applicant must *not* have been denied admission to the University of Florida College of Veterinary Medicine as a first-year student.
7. Applicants must have a letter approving transfer from their dean or associate dean.

University of Georgia

1. Priority is given to Georgia residents, followed by contract state residents, then all other applicants.
2. Applicants will be considered for entry in the second or third year.
3. Applications must include a letter of support written by a senior administrator of the school in which the applicant is currently enrolled.
4. All selection criteria for regular applicants apply to transfer applicants.
5. No individual is eligible for transfer who has been dismissed or is on probation at any other school or college for deficiency in scholarship or because of misconduct.

University of Illinois

1. Transfer students will only be considered for the beginning of the second year of veterinary medicine and only if transfer seats become available in that class.
2. All prerequisite science courses must be completed prior to the request for transfer.
3. Minimum grade requirements include:
   cumulative and science GPAs of 2.75 on a 4.00 scale (doesn't include veterinary work);
   semester GPA of 2.25 on a 4.00 scale (doesn't include veterinary work);
   results of the Graduate Record Examination General Test completed within the last two years.
4. Student must complete the same preveterinary coursework as required for all students accepted to the program.
5. Student must be in good academic standing.
6. To request transfer consideration, student must submit the "Notice of Interest to Transfer Form" found at
   http://www.cvm.uiuc.edu/asa/TransferInformation Form.pdf
7. To be considered for transfer, a student must present credentials for *preprofessional work* that fulfill the University of Illinois College of Veterinary Medicine requirements for first year entry.

8. All coursework must have been completed at a regionally accredited United States college or university.

Iowa State University

1. The applicant must have had essentially the same preveterinary coursework as required of Iowa State students and must have met the minimum qualifications of those admitted to the College of Veterinary Medicine.
2. The applicant must have completed the equivalent of all courses required of Iowa State University veterinary students beginning the academic term the applicant seeks to enter. Only credits earned at an AVMA accredited college of veterinary medicine will be considered for credit.
3. The applicant must have been in good standing throughout his or her entire period of enrollment in the school(s) of veterinary medicine in which the student is, or has been, enrolled. A letter to that effect from the dean(s) of the school(s) is required.
4. Space must be available.

Kansas State University

Acceptance of students for advanced standing is on recommendation of the Admissions Committee on a space-available basis.

Louisiana State University

1. There must be a vacancy in the class.
2. The curricula must be compatible.
3. The student must be in good academic standing with at least a 3.2 GPA in veterinary coursework at his/her present college.
4. Admission is limited to the second year of the program.
5. Each request for transfer is considered on a case-by-case basis.
6. To initiate the transfer process, the student must submit a formal letter of intent and all supporting documentation by March 1.

Michigan State University

1. Admission consideration is offered only to those current matriculants in professional veterinary curricula who believe that there are extenuating circumstances that would precipitate significant undue hardship if they continue at their current institution.
2. Applicants must also demonstrate quality academic performance throughout their professional school enrollment.
3. The curricula of the two schools must be sufficiently alike to allow a student to enter the second-year class without deficiencies in academic background.

4. All selection criteria for regular applicants apply to transfer applicants.
5. Priority is given to Michigan residents.
6. Space must be available.
7. AVMA accreditation of current school is considered.

University of Minnesota

1. Transfers are not allowed to any specific requested year or semester. The committee will place each applicant in the year or semester of the curriculum deemed appropriate after analysis of equivalency of the required courses involved.
2. No academic work or standing will be accepted from DVM curricula other than those deemed accredited ("AVMA accredited") by the American Veterinary Medical Association.
3. All applicants must be U.S. citizens, be holders of permanent resident alien visas, or have achieved landed immigrant status.
4. All applicants are required to have finished at least one full academic year at the institution from which transfer is requested and must be in good academic standing at the time of discontinuance according to written verification from the institution.
5. All applicants must document that not more than two calendar years have elapsed between discontinuance and application to our DVM program.
6. All applicants must have achieved a cumulative GPA of 3.00 (of 4.00) for the required courses at the initial institution.
7. All applicants must present suitable transcripts and course summary descriptions of all courses taken. These must be carried to the appropriate course coordinator in our curriculum, and each coordinator must certify in writing that the transfer courses satisfy our curricular specifications according to comparative criteria determined by each coordinator in discussion with the petitioner. The applicant is responsible for preparing a standard University of Minnesota Petition Form, obtaining the course instructor's dated signature, and returning it to the Office for Student Affairs and Admission. If equivalency is not certified, the course must be taken in our curriculum prior to the transfer to a specific veterinary class year.

Mississippi State University

Transfer students are accepted on a limited basis to fill vacancies in the freshman or sophomore class.

1. Any applicant must be in good academic standing, never have failed a course while in veterinary medical school, and never have been dismissed from a veterinary school.

2. Applicants considered for transfer admission will be required to attend an interview at Mississippi State University.
3. No transfer applicant is accepted at a point later than the second semester of the sophomore year. All veterinary medical students must complete at least two years at Mississippi State University to be eligible for a degree.
4. Students accepted into the phase 1 freshman or sophomore year are required to meet the College's current computer requirements.

For more information, contact the Student Affairs Assistant at the Office of Academic Affairs.

University of Missouri

1. Must be a vacancy in the class.
2. Will consider students who are U.S. citizens or holders of permanent alien visas and who have finished at least two years in a college of veterinary medicine that is AVMA accredited.
3. Students must be in good academic standing, and a letter of reference from the dean's office of the present college is required.

North Carolina State University

1. Must be a vacancy in the class.
2. Consideration by the Admission Committee on an individual basis.
3. Curricula must be compatible.
4. A letter from the dean of the current school certifying the applicant's academic standing.
5. Letter of recommendation from a faculty member at the original college.
6. Only accept transfers from AVMA accredited colleges.
7. At least 50% of DVM credit hours should be completed at North Carolina State in order to earn a North Carolina State degree.

Ohio State University

1. An opening must exist.
2. Student must be enrolled in an AVMA accredited college.
3. The curricula of the two schools must be sufficiently alike to allow the student to enter a class without deficiencies in his or her academic background.
4. Student must be in good academic standing in his or her present college and have a supporting letter from the Dean of Student and Academic Affairs to this effect.
5. Each request for transfer is considered on an individual basis, taking into account personal hardship, family situations, etc.
6. Must meet same prerequisite requirements as first-year applicants.

Oklahoma State University

1. A student will normally enter at the beginning of the fall semester, second year, regardless of his/her standing at the school from which he/she is transferring.
2. A student may be accepted only if a vacancy exists in the second-year class, fall semester.
3. Preference will be given to students from schools/colleges with AVMA accreditation.
4. Application deadline is April 15, with all requirements having been met prior to entry date.
5. Applications accepted only from students attending institutions that are accredited by an authentic accrediting agency.

Oregon State University

Admission of students with advanced standing is considered only in very specific and unique circumstances, and each case is considered on an individual basis.

University of Pennsylvania

1. An opening must exist.
2. Admission with Advanced Standing (AAS) is considered only from institutions that are accredited by the AVMA.
3. Student must initiate the process at his/her own institution. The Dean of Student Affairs at the college from which the student wants to transfer must understand the student's need for AAS and endorse it. The usual reasons endorsed are either medical or the desire to move nearer one's spouse.
4. If the Dean of Student Affairs approves, student must send detailed description of all coursework taken to date and simultaneously submit an application to the University of Pennsylvania's Admissions Committee. If the Admissions Committee accepts the credentials, it will compare coursework with that of the University of Pennsylvania and determine where in the curriculum the student might be placed.
5. If all criteria are met and space is available, AAS may be granted.
6. University of Pennsylvania cannot award a degree to a student who has completed less than 50% of graduation credits at Penn.

Purdue University

1. Positions must be available in the relevant class.
2. Student must have legitimate ties to the State of Indiana or extenuating/personal circumstance (e.g., transfer of spouse to Indiana for employment purposes).
3. Student must be in good academic standing in his/her present program.
4. Students must have completed 1–2 years of DVM courses with an exceptional academic record in those courses.
5. Veterinary medical curricula must be compatible.
6. Student must have support of the administration from the program in which he/she is currently enrolled.

University of Tennessee

Admission of students with advanced standing may be considered for unique circumstances on a case-by-case basis. Space must be available in the class and the professional curricula must reasonably match between the schools. The Admissions Committee will review applicants' credentials and interview those determined to best meet admission criteria. Admission is usually limited to the second semester of the first year of the professional curriculum. Students must be in good standing at their present college.

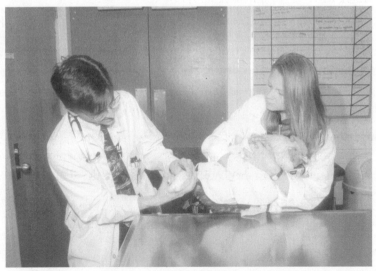

Colleges of veterinary medicine encourage teamwork. Here, students prepare to examine a chicken's injured foot. Photo by Phil Snow, courtesy of the University of Tennessee College of Veterinary Medicine.

Texas A & M University

Students requesting advanced standing must meet the following requirements:

1. Must have completed all previous professional veterinary courses in an AVMA accredited college of veterinary medicine.
2. Must have successfully completed the academic term preceding the semester into which student requests admission.
3. Must comply with all requirements for transfer into the university as described in the current catalog.
4. May request transfer only into the second through seventh semesters of the professional curriculum.
5. At the time of matriculation the student must certify by letter that he/she has not been convicted of crimes in the period from first enrollment in the college of veterinary medicine from which the student desires transfer until date of matriculation at Texas A&M University.
6. To request transfer consideration, the student must meet all requirements as posted on the College website at http://www.cvm.tamu.edu/dcvm/admissions.

Tufts University

Applicants from other veterinary schools are considered. Students with advanced standing are admitted if and when space becomes available in the second-year class. The application deadline is June 1 for the following September.

Washington State University

Admission of students with advanced standing is effected only in very specific and unique circumstances, and each case is considered on an individual basis.

University of Wisconsin

Admission of students with advanced standing is considered only in very specific and unique circumstances, and each case is considered on an individual basis.

INTERNATIONAL

University of Guelph

Applications for admission to advanced semesters will be considered from students who have been enrolled in DVM programs at other institutions, subject to the availability of spaces in the DVM Program and the academic standing of the candidate. When places are available, candidates may be asked to present themselves for an interview and may be asked to pass examinations on subject matter in the veterinary curriculum. Applicants are advised that vacancies are rare.

University of Prince Edward Island

Applicants who have completed all or portions of a veterinary medical program may apply for advanced standing to the second year of the DVM program. Applicants for advanced standing must present evidence of educational accomplishments and may be required to satisfactorily pass examinations in all of the courses for which they desire credit. Students admitted with advanced standing must begin the college year in September.

The candidate must file a formal application and may be interviewed by the Admissions Committee and possibly other faculty. Places for admission to the college with advanced standing are limited and depend on vacancies.

It is imperative that the Admissions Committee have detailed and translated summaries of veterinary medical academic programs and accomplishments for those seeking advanced placement from schools in foreign countries. Advanced-standing applications should be on file and completed as early as possible and no later than January 1.

University of Saskatchewan

Applications for admission with advanced standing will only be considered if a vacancy in the Year II class develops. Students applying for advanced standing must meet the normal residency requirements and must be enrolled in a program that has a compatible curriculum. Applicants are required to complete a formal application form and, dependant on their academic record, will be considered for an interview. Part of the interview will be an assessment of their current knowledge. Applicants will be required to submit a recent GRE score and, if English is not their first language, will also be required to submit a TOEFL score. Admission is not considered beyond the second year of the program.

APPLICATION AND ENROLLMENT DATA

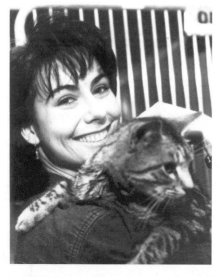

Job satisfaction: giving a little TLC during clinical rounds. Photo by Vivian Dixon, courtesy of University of Georgia College of Veterinary Medicine.

Table 1
Applicants to U.S. Colleges of Veterinary Medicine
by Residence, 2003–2006
VMCAS Data Only

State	2003	2004	2005	2006
Alberta	3	2	5	1
Alaska	8	7	7	6
Alabama	23	28	15	106
Arkansas	31	38	41	31
Arizona	75	92	78	81
British	4	6	6	3
California	335	329	367	557
Colorado	295	245	247	247
Connecticut	39	36	37	36
Washington, DC	5	3	4	5
Delaware	10	15	15	10
Florida	255	264	271	292
Foreign	18	18	22	16
Georgia	215	170	192	174
Guam	1	1	0	0
Hawaii	17	23	17	11
Iowa	11	16	17	112
Idaho	12	21	16	23
Illinois	216	212	227	232
Indiana	102	115	110	112
Kansas	17	17	19	20
Kentucky	33	39	41	124
Louisiana	152	142	132	124
Massachusetts	95	97	96	106
Manitoba	3	0	1	3
Maryland	105	102	79	106
Maine	11	14	16	18
Michigan	214	226	208	241
Minnesota	141	158	159	177
Missouri	20	22	21	20
Mississippi	64	58	56	56

Table 1 *(continued)*

State	2003	2004	2005	2006
Montana	27	28	20	28
North Carolina	201	175	197	224
North Dakota	21	14	20	23
Nebraska	12	23	26	47
New Hampshire	16	19	24	16
New Jersey	109	116	103	107
New Mexico	27	47	38	24
Nova Scotia	0	1	2	0
Nevada	23	23	24	26
New York	209	197	262	282
Ohio	90	123	79	102
Oklahoma	8	11	7	18
Ontario	5	9	10	16
Oregon	84	87	76	98
Pennsylvania	230	259	232	243
Puerto Rico	32	36	24	34
Rhode Island	10	10	9	9
South Carolina	75	67	57	66
South Dakota	18	8	16	14
Saskatchewan	0	0	0	1
Tennessee	121	101	132	138
U.S. Territories	1	0	1	1
Texas	101	139	139	132
Utah	29	33	33	32
Virginia	162	151	159	186
Virgin Islands	0	1	0	1
Vermont	10	10	11	8
Washington	61	58	51	48
Wisconsin	159	135	154	164
West Virginia	36	24	34	36
Wyoming	23	19	21	20

Table 2
Applicant Data for Classes 2003–2006
Applications by College
VMCAS Data Only

College	2003	2004	2005	2006
University of California, Davis	393	413	402	966**
Colorado State University	1,447	1,402	1475	1,482
Cornell University	437	464**	872	853
University of Florida	697	752	770	799
University of Georgia	607	547	566	524
University of Illinois	758	741	753	809
Louisiana State University	818	774	799	658
Michigan State University	1,010	1,015	884	1,008
University of Minnesota	643	655	751	916
Mississippi State University	378	363	381	369
North Carolina State University	518	513	564	600
Oklahoma State University	237	252	286	278
Oregon State University	661	668	630	663
University of Pennsylvania	1,110	1,216	1,246	1,291
Purdue University	630	611	590	583
University of Tennessee	269	464	768	763
Virginia-Maryland Regional College	761	745	785	872
Washington State University	562	617	647	641
University of Wisconsin	830	792	868	987
Auburn University	555	585	638	869**
University of Missouri	143	138	83	428
The Ohio State University	579	579	553	544
Iowa State University	464	510	553	647**
Kansas State University	315	425	498	603
University of Guelph-Ontario Veterinary College	43	80	104	96
University of PEI-Atlantic Veterinary College	213	190	186	187
University of Glasgow	225	193	172	181
Western University of Health Sciences	*	326	375	557
University of Edinburgh	*	101	132	169

* Was not a member of VMCAS in the year indicated.
** Indicates the year the college shifted from limited participation to full participation with VMCAS.

Table 3
Applicant Data for Classes 2003–2006
Age Distribution
VMCAS Data Only

Age	2003	2004	2005	2006
20	396	408	357	412
21	1,132	1,179	1,258	1,374
22	777	773	890	980
23	523	534	563	680
24	368	323	349	365
25–30	861	831	802	998
31–35	199	214	197	181
Older	193	191	165	204
Total	4,449	4,453	4,581	5,194

Table 4
Applicant Data for Classes 2003–2006
Gender Distribution
VMCAS Data Only

	2003 (% of pool)	2004 (% of pool)	2005 (% of pool)	2006 (% of pool)
Total Applicants	4,449	4,453	4,581	5,194
Applicants who identified gender	4,445	4,450	4,579	5,192
Females	3,545 (79.68%)	3,518 (79%)	3,682 80.38%	4,147 (79.84%)
Males	900 (20.23%)	932 (20.93%)	897 19.59%	1045 (20.12%)

% Change from:	2003/2004	2004/2005	2005/2006
Female	−0.76%	4.66%	12.63%
Male	3.56%	−3.76%	16.49%

Table 5

Applicant Data for Classes 2003–2006

	2003 (% responses)	
Number of Applicants	4449	
Number of applicants who identified themselves as part of 1 ethnic group	4107	92.31%
Number of applicants who identified themselves as part of 2 or more ethnic groups	96	2.16%
African-American/Black	75	1.69%
Spanish / Hispanic / Latino American	*	
No Spanish / Hispanic / Latino American	*	
Hispanic American	107	2.41%
Mexican / Mexican American / Chicano	40	0.899%
Puerto Rican	**	
Cuban	**	
Other Spanish / Hispanic / Latino American	**	
Other Latino / Spanish American	66	1.48%
American Indian / Alaskan Native	41	0.922%
Filipino / Filipino American	17	0.382%
Chinese / Chinese American	49	1.10%
East Indian	13	0.292%
Japanese / Japanese American	30	0.674%
Korean / Korean American	25	0.562%
Pacific Islander	10	0.225%
Other Asian	21	0.472%
Caucasian / Middle Eastern	3684	82.81%
Other	47	1.06%

Note: For the years 2003–2005 VMCAS categorized Spanish/Hispanic/ Latino as a race. However, according to the U.S. Census, it should be reported as an ethnicity. VMCAS has accordingly changed this category as follows:

   * in 2006 this category choice was moved to the heading of Ethnicity.

   ** was added as a specific ethnicity identifier.

   *** recategorized under ethnicity.

VMCAS fills between 59–75% of the seats of veterinary medical colleges. VMCAS statistics are seen as representative of the entire pool of applicants.

Ethnicity Distribution—% of Applicant Response
VMCAS Data Only

2004	(% responses)	2005	(% responses)	2006	(% responses)
4453		4581		5194	
4043	91.02%	4214	91.99%	4551	87.62%
103	2.31%	115	2.51%	3040	58.52%
72	1.62%	87	1.89%	82	1.58%
*		*		306	5.89%
*		*		2762	53.18%
106	2.38%	128	2.79%	***	
44	.988%	51	1.11%	94	1.81%
**		**		72	1.39%
**		**		30	0.578%
**		**		112	2.16%
56	1.26%	65	1.42%	***	
44	.988%	53	1.16%	63	1.21%.
13	0.292%	15	0.3275%	26	0.501%
74	1.66%	70	1.53%	74	1.42%
17	0.382%	18	0.392%	14	0.269%
48	1.08%	42	0.917%	52	1.001%
30	0.674%	23	0.502%	38	0.732%
12	0.269%	8	0.175%	8	0.154%
22	0.494%	23	0.502%	37	0.712%
3574	80.26%	3710	80.99%	3966	76.36%
51	1.15%	57	1.24%	64	1.23%

Table 6

TITLE IV

School	Perkins(NDSL) Loan		(Total) Stafford Loan		Un-Subsidized Stafford		Supplemental SLS & Plus	
	Amount	*No.*	*Amount*	*No.*	*Amount*	*No.*	*Amount*	*No.*
AUB	4,000	2	2,458,665	294	4,084,675	282		
UCD	490,601	257	3,134,358	380	3,010,352	321		
CSU	1,259,174	321	3,431,712	425				
COR	356,375	204	2,351,108	287	3,029,151	278		
FLA			2,248,901	273	3,466,994	278		
UGA	212,700	37	4,224,568	259	2,214,296	237		
ILL			2,502,530	319	2,662,847	252		
ISU			3,613,897	375	4,963,103	363		
KSU	157,550	91	2,250,753	272	2,242,449	250	35,653	7
LSU	275,750	37	1,841,607	61	1,908,028	60		
MSU	621,188	336	3,678,585	351	4,052,132	299		
MIN	106,153	24	2,421,532	293	5,563,504	273		
MIS			1,805,735	46	2,079,823	44		
UMO	610,419	50	1,850,979	58	1,648,460	51		
NCSU			1,825,608	229	3,306,048	236		
OSU			4,732,118	492	6,236,224	446		
OKL	71,665	16	1,996,837	239	2,532,591	215	62,129	12
ORE	67,800	38	1,022,216	61	523,643	56		
PENN	867,722	149	2,952,893	350	8,391,586	342		
PUR	7,100	4	3,546,433	472	1,929,773	255		
TENN	130,970	35	1,616,446	46	2,163,352	45		
TAMU	877,440	227	3,200,636	388	3,764,206	327		
TUF	139,200	36	2,022,291	241	5,838,294	235		
TUS			7,687,825	##	4,949,191	973	7,485,886	994
VMR	262	56	6,057,759	291	3,502,746	259		
WSU	750	1	2,534,229	315	3,975,223	283	3,224	1
WES	432,000	72	617,525	73	2,150,574	73		
WIS	1,493,313	257	2,240,193	271	3,158,494	250		

"No." = number of students

Sources of Financial Aid for 2003–2004 Academic Year

| TITLE IV | | TITLE VII | | | | | | | |
| Pell Grants | | HPSL | | HEAL | | LDS | | SDS | |
Amount	No.	Amount	No.	Amount	No.	Amount	No.	Amount	No.
		160,000	37						
		632,542	110			6,611	1		
		424,514	123						
		343,440	47						
		116,523	32						
		420,548	89			16,500	4		
		508,709	47						
32,950	13	484,590	79						
		901,696	117			52,650	16	27,037	18
		716,778	103						
		460,012	26						
		363,000	190			9,960	1	63,087	34
		134,027	18			20,880	16	52,143	27
		1,147,795	139						
		450,780	37						
59,646	17								
		9,900	4			20,000	8		
		140,600	37						
3,494,300	1,084								
		202,000	67						
1,450	1	521,019	67						

Table 7

School	Tuition & Fees Res	NR	Room & Board Res	NR	Books & Equipment Res	NR	Personal Res	NR
AUB	9,778	28,898	6,692	6,692	2,250	2,250	2,424	2,424
UCD	18,685	30,930	10,510	10,510	1,409	1,409	1,842	1,842
CSU	11,525	35,724	6,045	6,045	1,154	1,154	1,421	1,421
COR	20,500	29,000	7,650	7,650	900	900	4,798	4,798
FLA	13,092	35,662	9,380	9,380	1,486	1,486	740	740
UGA	10,196	10,196	6,006	6,006	1,000	1,000	1,740	1,740
ILL	14,392	34,856	8,550	8,550	1,150	1,150	2,020	2,020
ISU	10,986	27,948	7,700	7,700	989	989	2,096	2,096
KSU	12,085	31,888	7,576	7,576	861	861	1,643	1,643
LSU	11,333	28,233	11,000	11,000	2,000	2,000	2,200	2,200
MSU	14,834	31,034	8,550	8,550	1,382	1,382	1,800	1,800
MIN	17,342	33,131	5,986	5,986	1,588	1,588	1,642	1,642
MIS	8,205	24,705	7,250	7,250	8,325	8,325		3,113
UMO	14,360	27,590	8,210	8,210	1,350	1,350	5,510	5,510
NCSU	9,445	32,208	8,310	8,310	2,002	2,002	1,604	1,604
OSU	16,386	41,610	6,048	6,048	1,854	1,854	1,056	1,056
OKL	10,890	27,030	6,430	6,430	900	900	2,100	2,100
ORE	14,790	28,263	6,786	6,786	1,200	1,200	2,181	2,181
PENN	28,214	33,474	12,570	12,570	1,000	1,000	4,500	4,500
PUR	12,596	30,364	7,020	7,020	1,272	1,272	1,040	1,040
TENN	10,176	28,396	7,400	7,400	2,536	2,536	2,880	2,880
TAMU	11,371	22,171	9,306	9,306	1,595	1,595	2,652	2,652
TUF	28,310	33,244			150	150		
TUS	13,730	13,730	5,249	5,249	1,786	5,352	1,714	3,428
VMR	12,867	29,139	6,000	6,000	1,000	1,000	1,000	1,000
WSU	12,654	31,212	10,000	10,000	1,900	1,900		1,434
WES		30,755		10,380		1,575		3,170
WIS	15,882	23,916	6,940	6,940	1,110	1,110	1,860	1,860
US Avg	14,245	29,118	7,814	7,909	1,635	1,760	2,186	2,294
ONT	2,272	21,457						
MON	3,200		7,000		1,100			
PEI	8,189	44,579	6,900	6,900	3,000	3,000	2,000	2,000
SKW	7,002		6,500		3,100			

NR = Non-resident; refers to all out-of-state/at-large applicants

DVM Student Tuition and Fees—First Year (Class of 2008)

Transportation		Health		Other		TOTAL EXPENSES	
Res	NR	Res	NR	Res	NR	Res	NR
1,574	1,574	879	879			23,597	42,717
1,202	1,202	1,446	1,446			35,094	47,339
567	567	970	970			21,682	45,881
		1,202	1,202			35,050	43,550
410	410	1,570	1,570	1,210	1,210	27,888	50,458
					16,900	18,942	35,842
470	800	466	466			27,048	47,842
1,218	1,218	846	846			23,835	40,797
1,700	1,700	1,495	1,495	1,791	1,791	27,151	46,954
1,650	1,650	800	800			28,983	45,883
1,188	1,188	1,226	1,226			28,980	45,180
750	750	1,238	1,238	2,000	2,000	30,546	46,335
3,113					26,893	43,393	
						29,430	42,660
1,604	1,604					22,965	45,728
1,536	1,536	1,008	1,008	2,187	2,187	30,075	55,299
1,560	1,560					21,880	38,020
				250	250	25,207	38,680
		2,072	2,072			48,356	53,616
1,340	1,660					23,268	41,356
2,050	2,050					25,042	43,262
692	692					25,616	36,416
	185	185	25	25	28,670	33,604	
428	921	857	857	1,571	1,217	25,335	30,754
750	750	580	580	800	800	22,997	39,269
1,434	1,250	1,250	474	474	27,712	46,270	
	3,085		648		375	0	49,988
410	410	1,310	1,310	450	450	27,962	35,996
1,221	1,358	1,078	1,055	1,076	2,307	26,436	43,325
						2,272	21,457
						11,300	0
1,000	2,400	179	679	2,700	2,700	23,968	62,258
2,136				2,190		20,928	0

Table 8
Summary of Non-DVM Degrees Awarded (Classes 2003–2004)

School	BS			MS			PhD			**Other		
	Total	Min.*	%Min.	Total	Min.*	%Min	Total	Min.*	%Min.	Total	Min.*	%Min.
AUB				7	1	14.3%	4	1	25.0%			
UCD	9	2	22.2%	18	9	50.0%	16	8	50.0%	2		0.0%
CSU	85	14	16.5%	96	8	8.3%	15	3	20.0%			
COR				1	1	100.0%	13	7	53.8%			
FLA				6	4	66.7%	7	4	57.1%			
UGA				7	2	28.6%	14	3	21.4%	2	1	50.0%
ILL	90	8	8.9%	12	3	25.0%	7	2	28.6%			
ISU				12	4	33.3%	11	2	18.2%			
KSU				1		0.0%	3	1	33.3%			
LSU				6	2	33.3%	7	3	42.9%			
MSU	51	2	3.9%	12	7	58.3%	8	5	62.5%			
MIN				13	1	7.7%	19		0.0%	32	1	3.1%
MIS				8		0.0%	1		0.0%			
UMO				8	2	25.0%	9	5	55.6%			
NCSU				1		0.0%	5	2	40.0%	2		0.0%

| | BS | | | MS | | | PhD | | | **Other | | |
School	Total	Min.*	%Min.	Total	Min.*	%Min.	Total	Min.*	%Min.	Total	Min.*	%Min.
OSU				19	2	10.5%	15	6	40.0%	24		0.0%
OKL				4	3	75.0%	5	4	80.0%			
ORE				1		0.0%						
PENN							9	2	22.2%			
PUR	29	1	3.4%	7	2	28.6%	6	4	66.7%	29	1	3.4%
TENN				1		0.0%	3	2	66.7%			
TAMU	1986	463	23.3%	13	3	23.1%	22	6	27.3%			
TUF				9	2	22.2%						
TUS				1	1	100.0%						
VMR				11	1	9.1%	4		0.0%			
WSU	23	3	13.0%	5	1	20.0%	13	7	53.8%			
WES												
WIS				6		0.0%	8	2	25.0%			
ONT												
MON	1		0.0%	18	6	33.3%	5	1	20.0%			
PEI				5		0.0%	2		0.0%			
SKW				17		0.0%	3		0.0%			

* Min = minority students
** Other = excludes DVM degree

Table 9
DVM Student Attrition (Classes 2004–2007)

School	*CAUCASIAN YR1	YR2	YR3	YR4	TOTAL	MINORITY YR1	YR2	YR3	YR4	TOTAL	GRAND TOTAL
AUB		1			1					0	1
UCD					0					0	0
CSU					0					0	0
COR	3				3	1				1	4
FLA	2				2		1			1	3
UGA	1			1	2					0	2
ILL	4	1			5					0	5
ISU	5	3	2		10					0	10
KSU					0					0	0
LSU	2	1			3					0	3
MSU	2				2					0	2
MIN					0					0	0
MIS	6	1		1	8					0	8
UMO		3			3					0	3
NCSU			1		1					0	1
OSU			1	3	4					0	4
OKL	2	2		1	5					0	5
ORE	1				1					0	1
PENN	3				3					0	3
PUR	3	3		1	7					0	7
TENN	1	3			4	1				1	5
TAMU	2	3			5	1				1	6
TUF	3				3					0	3
TUS					0	2	1			3	3
VMR					0					0	0
WSU	2	3	1		6	1				1	7
WES					0					0	0
WIS				1	1	1				1	2
US Total	42	24	5	8	79	7	2	0	0	9	88
ONT	1	2	1	2	6					0	6
MON	1	2	3	1	7					0	7
PEI		1			1					0	1
SKW					0					0	0
Can. Total	2	5	4	3	14	0	0	0	0	0	14
Grand Total	44	29	9	11	93	7	2	0	0	9	102

*Canadian institutions do not all report ethnic identity. For the purpose of this table, students may be reported under the Caucasian column.

Table 10
Reasons for DVM Student Attrition (Classes 2004–2007)

School	CAUCASIAN Low Grades	Other	Total	MINORITY Low Grades	Other	Total	GRAND TOTAL
AUB		1	1			0	1
UCD			0			0	0
CSU			0			0	0
COR	1	2	3	1		1	4
FLA	2		2		1	1	3
UGA	1	1	2			0	2
ILL	1	4	5			0	5
ISU	8	2	10			0	10
KSU			0			0	0
LSU	2	1	3			0	3
MSU		2	2			0	2
MIN			0			0	0
MIS	6	2	8			0	8
UMO	3		3			0	3
NCSU	1		1			0	1
OSU	2	2	4			0	4
OKL	2	3	5			0	5
ORE	1		1			0	1
PENN	1	2	3			0	3
PUR	1	6	7			0	7
TENN	2	2	4	1		1	5
TAMU	5		5		1	1	6
TUF		3	3			0	3
TUS			0	1	2	3	3
VMR			0			0	0
WSU	2	4	6		1	1	7
WES			0			0	0
WIS	1		1		1	1	2
US Total	42	37	79	3	6	9	88
ONT		6	6			0	6
MON	1	6	7			0	7
PEI		1	1			0	1
SKW			0			0	0
Can. Total	1	13	14	0	0	0	14
Grand Total	43	50	93	3	6	9	102

*Canadian institutions do not all report ethnic identity. For the purposes of this table, students may be reported under the Caucasian column.

Table 11
DVM Student Raw Test Scores—First Year (Class of 2008)

School	Mean GRE Verbal	Mean GRE Quantitative	Mean GRE Analytical	Mean Advanced Biology	Mean VCAT	Mean MCAT	Mean Other	Other Tests Defined
AUB	489	621						
UCD	569	711	5					
CSU	517	639	646					
COR	590	730						
FLA	526	675						
UGA	526	648	4.7	611				
ILL	496	636						
ISU	479	631						
KSU	501	648	667					
LSU	497	642						
MSU	510	650				23		
MIN	540	650						
MIS	426	542						
UMO				413	94	22		
NCSU	515	632	667.41				5	NEW ANALYTICAL
OSU					75			

176

School	Mean GRE Verbal	Mean GRE Quantitative	Mean GRE Analytical	Mean Advanced Biology	Mean VCAT	Mean MCAT	Mean Other	Other Tests Defined
OKL	448	576		542				
ORE	485	610	4.5					
PENN	570	710						
PUR	506	657	656					
TENN	492	612	4.42					
TAMU	494	664	4.67					
TUF	620	700	5					
TUS								
VMR	550	675	5					
WSU								
WES	486	633	623					
WIS	544	675	4.8					

Table 12

School	Mean Pre-Vet GPA	Grade Scale	Mean Age	Years of Pre-Professional Prep (Number of Students with ...)					
				Mean Yrs. of Prep.	2yr	3yr	4yr	5yr	6(+)yr
AUB	3.46	A = 4.00	23.00	4.30		19	39	21	12
UCD	3.50	A = 4.00	26.00	4.00	4	17	46	26	29
CSU	3.55	A = 4.00	25.00	4.82	3	11	25	38	56
COR	3.73	A = 4.00	23.00	5.00		5	69	4	7
FLA	3.56	A = 4.00	25.10	4.65		7	36	17	22
UGA	3.53	A = 4.00	24.40						
ILL	3.48	A = 4.00	25.10	5.90	1	5	37	24	29
ISU	3.51	A = 4.00	23.50	4.00		18	74	11	4
KSU	3.50	A = 4.00	23.90	4.60		15	48	18	22
LSU	3.78	A = 4.00	23.73	3.84	19	14	29	10	14
MSU	3.54	A = 4.00	23.83		6	14	79	7	22
MIN	3.48	A = 4.00	26.00	4.50		18	41	15	151
MIS	3.47	A = 4.00	23.00	4.00	2	25	40	3	2
UMO	3.63	A = 4.00	23.00		1	23	43		2
NCSU	3.55	A = 4.00	24.50	4.00	1		72		3
OSU	3.59	A = 4.00	23.73	4.50		17	91	18	14
OKL	3.42	A = 4.00	24.00	4.70		9	26	26	20
ORE	3.48	A = 4.00	24.96	5.57		2	19	15	131
PENN	3.54	A = 4.00	24.40	4.50			90	10	8
PUR	3.68	A = 4.00	22.00	4.00	2	17	37	8	3
TENN	3.49	A = 4.00	24.00	4.40	3	9	31	10	17
TAMU	3.64	A = 4.00	23.00	4.50		12	41	52	24
TUF	3.59	A = 4.00	27.00						
TUS	3.24	A = 4.00	22.70	4.30		5	36	12	5
VMR	3.55	A = 4.00	23.92	4.20	2	4	60	17	8
WSU	3.62	A = 4.00	25.00	4.20	1	11	46	37	6
WES	3.25	A = 4.00	28.00						
WIS	3.43	A = 4.00	25.00	4.00		14	43	11	2
US Avg	3.53		24.31	4.46	4	13	48	18	14
ONT									
MON			20.40	2.80	43	21	9	4	3
PEI	3.30	A = 4.00	24.00	4.60			15	5	4
SKW	6.14			3.99	9	17	23	14	7

Profile of Professional First Year DVM Students (Class of 2008)

Number of Students with Degrees

No Degree Complete	BS/BA	MS/MA	PhD
12	71	8	
9	113	7	2
1	109	21	1
5	76	3	1
72	16		
7	87	4	
13	88	5	
12	87	5	
22	74	7	
47	36	1	
20	79	7	2
18	65	5	1
20	43	9	
23	43	2	
	72	2	
19	116	5	
34	47	1	
	44	4	1
	100	8	
31	36		
8	62	2	
91	38	3	
1	71	7	1
2	56		
6	80	5	
27	68	4	
	69	9	1
14	54	11	2
19	70	6	1
43	58	9	1
74	5	1	
	24		
28	42		

Table 13

School	African Amer.		Hispanic		Asian		Pacific Islander		Native American		Alaskan Native		Multi-Ethnic	
	m	f	m	f	m	f	m	f	m	f	m	f	m	f
AUB	2	4	2	1	2	1	0	0	1	1	0	0	0	0
UCD	1	1	4	18	10	38	0	0	0	1	0	0	1	10
CSU	0	0	6	19	6	21	0	0	1	4	0	0	0	12
COR	3	16	5	23	2	16	0	0	0	6	0	0	0	0
FLA	3	5	3	22	2	6	0	1	0	0	0	0	0	0
UGA	0	6	1	7	1	7	0	0	1	0	0	0	2	2
ILL	1	1	1	0	0	0	0	0	0	0	0	0	0	0
ISU	0	0	2	1	0	6	0	0	0	0	0	0	0	0
KSU	1	0	1	4	1	6	0	0	0	0	0	0	0	0
LSU	1	3	5	9	2	4	0	0	0	0	0	0	0	3
MSU	0	3	6	14	3	11	0	0	2	5	0	0	0	0
MIN	0	0	1	1	0	9	0	0	0	1	0	0	1	0
MIS	2	2	1	3	0	3	0	0	0	0	0	0	0	0
UMO	0	4	1	3	1	3	0	0	1	0	0	0	0	0
NCSU	0	4	1	1	1	5	0	0	0	2	0	0	0	0
OSU	0	1	4	3	4	7	0	0	0	0	0	0	0	0
OKL	0	3	3	6	0	3	0	0	16	10	0	0	0	0
ORE	0	0	0	2	0	2	0	0	0	0	0	0	1	2
PENN	0	5	2	7	3	15	0	0	0	1	0	0	0	0
PUR	1	1	1	7	0	3	0	2	0	0	0	0	0	0
TENN	0	2	0	1	0	1	0	0	0	0	0	0	0	0
TAMU	2	2	7	22	3	10	0	0	1	0	0	0	0	0
TUF	2	0	0	1	2	11	0	0	0	2	0	0	0	0
TUS	28	64	9	19	1	5	0	0	0	2	0	0	0	3
VMR	1	9	1	2	1	5	0	4	0	3	0	0	0	0
WSU	0	0	2	5	2	7	0	0	0	0	0	2	0	0
WES	0	0	1	13	1	17	0	0	0	1	0	0	0	0
WIS	2	6	2	10	1	6	0	0	0	0	0	0	0	0
US	50	142	72	224	49	228	0	7	23	39	0	2	5	32
ONT	0	0	0	0	0	0	0	0	0	0	0	0	0	0
MON	4	0	1	0	1	1	0	0	0	0	0	0	0	0
PEI	0	0	0	0	0	0	0	0	0	0	0	0	0	0
SKW	0	0	0	0	0	0	0	0	0	0	0	0	0	0
Can	4	0	1	0	1	1	0	0	0	0	0	0	0	0
Total	54	142	73	224	50	229	0	7	23	39	0	2	5	32

*N/A - Not available; Canadian institutions do not all report ethnic identity.

Total DVM Student Enrollment by Ethnic Identity (Classes 2005–2008)

Other Minority		Minority Total			N/A*		Foreign National		Caucasian		Grand Total		
m	f	m	f	all	m	f	m	f	m	f	m	f	all
0	1	7	8	15	0	0	0	0	119	235	126	243	369
6	13	22	81	103	5	23	1	0	65	299	93	403	496
0	0	13	56	69	21	37	0	1	85	322	119	416	535
0	0	10	61	71	0	0	0	3	56	206	66	270	336
0	0	8	34	42	0	0	0	0	61	225	69	259	328
1	7	6	29	35	0	0	0	0	81	250	87	279	366
3	18	5	19	24	1	0	0	1	82	292	88	312	400
0	1	2	8	10	9	18	0	3	97	269	108	298	406
0	0	3	10	13	0	0	1	3	140	277	144	290	434
1	0	9	19	28	0	0	0	1	71	233	80	253	333
0	1	11	34	45	0	0	2	2	52	318	65	354	419
0	0	2	11	13	0	0	0	3	55	271	57	285	342
0	0	3	8	11	0	0	1	0	79	141	83	149	232
0	6	3	16	19	0	0	0	0	54	184	57	200	257
0	3	2	15	17	0	6	0	0	45	233	47	254	301
0	0	8	11	19	0	0	0	0	117	410	125	421	546
0	0	19	22	41	0	0	0	0	71	184	90	206	296
0	0	1	6	7	0	0	0	0	31	132	32	138	170
3	8	8	36	44	1	1	0	6	86	304	95	347	442
0	0	2	13	15	0	0	0	0	55	190	57	203	260
0	0	0	4	4	1	2	0	0	50	211	51	217	268
0	0	13	34	47	1	2	0	0	122	339	136	375	511
0	0	4	14	18	0	0	1	5	61	231	66	250	316
0	5	38	98	136	0	0	2	0	27	62	67	160	227
0	1	3	24	27	0	0	0	0	60	272	63	296	359
0	0	4	14	18	0	0	0	0	87	229	91	243	334
0	0	2	31	33	1	17	1	2	18	90	22	140	162
0	0	5	22	27	0	0	0	1	71	214	76	237	313
14	**64**	**213**	**738**	**951**	**40**	**106**	**9**	**31**	**1998**	**6623**	**2260**	**7498**	**9758**
0	0	0	0	0	73	348	4	5	0	0	77	353	430
0	1	6	2	8	0	0	6	23	66	261	78	286	364
0	0	0	0	0	28	123	17	72	0	0	45	195	240
0	0	0	0	0	0	0	0	0	0	0	0	0	0
0	1	6	2	8	101	471	27	100	66	261	200	834	1034
14	**65**	**219**	**740**	**959**	**141**	**577**	**36**	**131**	**2064**	**6884**	**2460**	**8332**	**10792**